THE HEALING ENIGMA

DEMYSTIFYING HOMEOPATHY

VINTON MCCABE

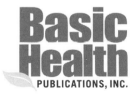

Basic Health
PUBLICATIONS, INC.

The information contained in this book is based upon the research and personal and professional experiences of the author. It is not intended as a substitute for consulting with your physician or other healthcare provider. Any attempt to diagnose and treat an illness should be done under the direction of a healthcare professional.

The publisher does not advocate the use of any particular healthcare protocol but believes the information in this book should be available to the public. The publisher and author are not responsible for any adverse effects or consequences resulting from the use of the suggestions, preparations, or procedures discussed in this book. Should the reader have any questions concerning the appropriateness of any procedures or preparation mentioned, the author and the publisher strongly suggest consulting a professional healthcare advisor.

Basic Health Publications, Inc.
28812 Top of the World Drive
Laguna Beach, CA 92651
949-715-7327 • www.basichealthpub.com

Library of Congress Cataloging-in-Publication Data

McCabe, Vinton.
    The healing enigma : demystifying homeopathy / by Vinton McCabe.
      p. cm.
    Includes index.
    ISBN-13: 978-1-59120-071-0
    ISBN-10: 1-59120-071-7
    1. Homeopathy. I. Title.
RX71.M328 2006
615.5'32—dc22

                                              2006015744

Editor: Cheryl Hirsch
Typesetting/Book design: Gary A. Rosenberg
Cover design: Mike Stromberg

Printed in the United States of America

10   9   8   7   6   5   4   3   2   1

"The highest ideal of cure is the rapid, gentle, and permanent restoration of health."

—SAMUEL HAHNEMANN
IN THE ORGANON OF MEDICINE

Contents

PART THREE

Healing

Acknowledgments

There are three people who must be thanked for their assistance in the creation of this book.

First, I must thank Julian Winston, a homeopathic historian and educator without peer, who, sadly, passed away soon after reading through the manuscript for this book and offering his insight, advice, and corrections where needed. Whether we agreed upon a common viewpoint or not, I always found it to be quite impossible not to both respect and enjoy Julian. Because he was nearly as crabby as I am. And because he was always honest, and nearly always correct—a formidable combination. I thank him for being a guardian angel for this book and dedicate it to him.

Second, I wish to thank Wenda Brewster O'Reilly, who so kindly once more gave me permission to quote from the recent translation of Hahnemann's the *Organon of Medicine* that she edited. Wenda is the rarest of humans, a true scholar who has a mind that is at once wide open and razor sharp. I thank her for giving this book the gift of Hahnemann's wisdom in the best and clearest of translations.

Finally, I want to thank my own homeopathic practitioner, Tina Zigo, N.D. Not only because she took the time and trouble to read this book in manuscript and not roll her eyes too often, but also because she has, for me, been both a true physician and a true friend.

Introduction

It was exactly half my lifetime ago now, in the summer of 1980, that I first heard the word "homeopathy." I heard the word at a lecture given in a health spa in Westport, Connecticut. On first hearing, the word meant little to me—in fact, I placed it, along with crystals, auras, and Sufi dancing, in the category of vaguely amusing things that affluent people will come up with when they have too much time on their hands.

Back in those dark ages, about twenty-five years ago now, there was very little information available on the subject. The Internet had yet to be born and what few books you could find on the subject were either paperback originals with all the literary quality of telephone books or musty antiques that had been self-published a century ago and that had been quickly sold when someone's quirky uncle or grandfather died.

I bought a couple of these paperbacks and soon knew a list of ten or twelve remedy names and had a full understanding of the two whole sentences that were listed about each. I also had a new understanding of medicine, one based in the perhaps simplistic messages that these books had to offer: homeopathy good, allopathy bad.

When a physical need presented itself, I decided to try homeopathy and see if it worked. I was living in the hot sweaty climate of south Texas at the time, and driving around in a '64 Volkswagen Beetle that had no air conditioning.* Because of the heat and dust, I found myself with a case of very bad acne even though I was in my late twenties. I remembered the lecture that I had heard in Westport a few years before, and, since I had seen homeopathic remedies at the local health-food store, I decided to try one and see if it worked. I bought the remedy Sulphur because one of my books

---

* Once I found myself and my Beetle entrapped by a herd of cattle that broke through their fence and surrounded me like one of the gangs in *West Side Story*, but that has nothing to do with homeopathy. It did, however, make me yearn for Connecticut.

said, in the two sentences that it dedicated to the remedy, that it was very good for skin conditions, although it didn't mention acne specifically.

I took the remedy for a few days. At first I didn't notice much of anything. Then, after a couple more days, my skin got so much worse, turning bright red and breaking out all over the place. And I found that I was hotter, sweatier, and thirstier than I had been before.

I immediately stopped taking the remedy and swore that I would never do that again. In a few days, the skin flare-up settled down and I just put up with the skin condition until I moved back to Connecticut, where I belonged. What I hadn't known about Connecticut before I left was that it was a veritable hotbed of homeopathy, one of three states in the country that actually allowed the practice of homeopathy within its borders. From there, let's just say that homeopathy got bitch-slapped into my life by a series of personal health crises.

But back to Texas and my skin condition for a moment. You see, when I took that remedy Sulphur, I knew so little about homeopathy and what it truly was and what its impact could be that I didn't realize that I had actually, through sheer luck, happened onto a remedy that could have done me some good, and that the flare-up of my skin condition was really a signal that the remedy was working. The remedy was clearing my skin by pushing out the blemishes very quickly. Had I waited it out and kept with the remedy I would have likely found a distinct improvement within the next few days.

But I didn't know what I was doing. Either in selecting the remedy or in taking it.

In this way, my first experience with a homeopathic remedy was very similar to that of thousands of other Americans who try a remedy—often Arnica for an injury or Oscillicoccinum for flu—and have one of two negative results. Either they find that their symptoms mysteriously flare up and actually grow worse after taking the remedy, or they find that nothing whatsoever happens. Either way, they tend to think that homeopathy is a bad thing, even though they have never actually experienced homeopathy, only the effects of a badly chosen or badly used homeopathic remedy.

Like most of us who get involved with homeopathy in this country, I had to just jump in with very little information and hope for the best. At least I started with a benign condition like acne. Over the years, I have seen others that, let us say, were not so prudent. I have seen totally unskilled and unknowledgeable people jump in with conditions like cancer—life-threatening conditions—or allergies or learning disabilities—chronic, complex conditions—and I have seen the disastrous results.

Over the next twenty-odd years, as I learned more and more about homeopathy in both its philosophy and practice, as I taught homeopathy in class after class to thousands of laypeople and medical professionals alike in many different parts of this country, I saw so many people who came to homeopathy for one very simple reason:

they were desperate. Sometimes they were ill themselves, but more often someone they loved was very ill. Sometimes the people coming into the classes came to learn and to learn as much as they could. They truly wanted to understand the philosophy of homeopathy first, to grasp its history, and then turn their attention to its art and practice as well. But far more often they came to one class or two. Then they would join the line to speak with me after class in order to ask me one of two questions. They would either want to explain their challenge in one or two sentences and then ask me what remedy would cure everything or they would ask me for the secret name of the very best homeopath in the world.

When I first taught, or more accurately, when I was learning while teaching (to be honest, in the beginning I was using one of my paperbacks as a text and trying my best to stay a page ahead of my students), I would often find that I could not refuse to try and help the person standing in front of me and asking for help. They would seem to be in so much pain, with a beloved child or parent or partner or pet who was suffering so. I would try once again to guess—and, in truth, that's all you can do when you only have a sentence or two to work with—a remedy that might help. Or I would tell them the name of a practitioner who I thought could help them.

But I wised up fast. After a few came back, red faced with rage, to tell me that the remedy didn't cure everything or that they didn't like that practitioner, I came to understand that all I could do is offer the best information I could and then let them take it from there. All I could hope is that they would put enough time in to either learn to take and manage the case on their own or to know what questions to ask, what skills to expect in selecting their own homeopath. It became my goal not to teach each one to become a homeopath, but, instead to teach them to become wise consumers of homeopathy.

When you teach a subject like this one, you have to keep your goal clear. It was never my goal to train practitioners or to become a practitioner or to sell remedies. It was my goal to make information that had heretofore not been available to the public or available to anyone who wanted it. This was the information that had to do with the actual nature of homeopathy, in the manner in which the German physician Samuel Hahnemann himself codified it more than two centuries ago. This was the information of what could and could not be expected from homeopathic medicine, how and why it worked, and how it must be practiced if it is to be safe and effective. The same information that is contained within the pages of this book.

If we can jump ahead twenty-five years now to the present, it seems to me that the need for education remains just as great as it ever was. And ironically a great deal of the problem now has to do with homeopathy's popularity, rather than the obscurity that plagued it a generation ago.

Now there are hundreds of websites dedicated to homeopathy, hundreds of books on the subject, study groups, formal classes that, in many cases, cost a fortune to join, and diplomas and certificates galore, many of which offer no legal right whatsoever to actually practice homeopathy. There are clubs and organizations by the dozen and, at least here in Connecticut, many more practitioners than we need. One of my very first teachers, an author and practitioner named S. K. Bannerjea, once told our class that homeopathy was so popular in his native India that, if you threw a rock into a crowd, you were likely to strike a homeopath. So many times in the past few years, I have been sorely tempted to throw rocks into crowds right here, in the hopes that I could lower the practitioner to patient average here at home.

We are still living in a world that is largely ignorant on the topic of homeopathy. People still seem to be unable to differentiate between herbal and homeopathic medicines. They still mistakenly use the word "homeopathic" for any form of natural medicine. And they still don't seem to get it that homeopathy and allopathy just don't work in the same way, and that you can't expect the same results from these very different processes.

However, we are no longer suffering from too little information as we were a generation ago. No, now we are suffering from too much *bad* information. Too many websites that just plain have it wrong. And too many "practitioners" and "educators," who in recent years came to homeopathy, and seem themselves to be confused as to the nature of homeopathy and its practice. And computer software has made it all too easy for these guys to just type in the symptoms and let the machine do all the work. Pity that they haven't realized that these software packages can't do all the work, that they still have to know how to take cases, and they actually have to type in real, useful information in order to get real and useful results. Pity that they haven't learned, as American homeopath James Tyler Kent taught his students decades ago, that homeopathic remedies used allopathically act in the patient's system like allopathic drugs. They bastardize their use of homeopathic remedies and get allopathic results and haven't the skill to understand why.

Hahnemann, Kent, and the other fathers of homeopathy had a word for such practitioners. They called them "half-homeopaths" because they practiced a supposed form of homeopathy that failed to follow the rules of homeopathic treatment. But anything that attempts to blend the philosophy of allopathy with the practice of homeopathy invariably falls into the chasm that lies between the two.

We ask a great deal from those who practice homeopathy.* This is because homeopathy is a very complex subject for study. It requires an understanding of the nature

* For our purposes in this book, the word "practitioner" will apply equally to those medical professionals who use homeopathic remedies and to those laypeople who make use of remedies for themselves and their loved ones.

of illness and health and the journey that must be traveled between these two poles of the human condition. It also demands an understanding of the nature of medicine and its ability or lack thereof to move the patient from illness toward health. It also requires an understanding of the philosophy of homeopathy—a philosophy that was some two thousand years in the shaping before Samuel Hahnemann ever coined the word "homeopathy" in order to codify what so many others had attempted beforehand. Finally, it requires an understanding of the remedies that comprise the homeopathic pharmacy (and there are thousands) and the ability to recognize the remedy need that any given patient is displaying "on the hoof."

Because homeopathy is such a complex subject, it is one that no one, not even Hahnemann himself, can fully master in a lifetime. To the end of his days, Hahnemann was rewriting his *Organon**, always including new ideas, new possibilities, not only of new additions to the homeopathic pharmacy, but also as to the nature of homeopathy itself. In the two hundred years since Hahnemann, hundreds of others have contributed their thoughts and ideas as to the nature of homeopathy and its practice. Some have, in my opinion, crystallized the truth of homeopathy, while others—sometimes the most celebrated of homeopaths—have moved us further away from the truth. Like politics, like religion, homeopathy is a subject that seems to encourage debate, especially between its proponents. Further it is a subject that we can only test over a lifetime of study and use, learning and grasping a bit more understanding as we go.

Therefore, no one book on the subject of homeopathy can ever tell you the whole story, the whole truth. Indeed, no bookshelf of books can do that. Each can only tell you *their* story of homeopathy. The facts as they know them, as they were passed on to them, and as they have experienced them. Their own truths, their own experiences.

This book is about what I have learned about homeopathy over the years, about what the study of this subject has taught me. It is the truth as I have experienced it, as I know it.

I pass this truth on to you.

---

* The *Organon of Medicine* was Samuel Hahnemann's magnum opus. Instead of writing many different books on the subject of his expertise, as most would do, Hahnemann instead took his *Organon* through six separate editions (1810, 1819, 1824, 1829, 1833, and 1842), each of which changed and evolved in content even as Hahnemann's own homeopathic philosophy evolved and developed. In this way, the *Organon* can be considered almost a living creature, maturing and changing along with its author. The word "organon" by the way means "organ" or "system." It is a name given to the major work by an expert in which he puts down into writing the fundamentals of his topic. In this case, as the fundamentals grew, so did the *Organon*.

PART ONE

Medicine

"You do solemnly swear, each by whatever he or she holds most sacred:
That you will be loyal to the Profession of Medicine and just and generous
to its members. That you will lead your lives and practice your art in
uprightness and honor.

"That into whatsoever house you shall enter, it shall be for the good
of the sick to the utmost of your power, your holding yourselves far aloof
from wrong, from corruption, from the tempting of others to vice.

"That you will exercise your art solely for the cure of your patients,
and will give no drug, perform no operation, for a criminal purpose,
even if solicited, far less suggest it.

"That whatsoever you shall see or hear of the lives of men or women
which is not fitting to be spoken, you will keep inviolably secret.

"These things do you swear. Let each bow the head in sign of
acquiescence. And now, if you will be true to this, your oath,
may prosperity and good repute be ever yours; the opposite,
if you shall prove yourselves forsworn."

—A MODERN VARIATION ON THE ANCIENT HIPPOCRATIC OATH,
APPROVED BY THE AMERICAN MEDICAL ASSOCIATION

CHAPTER ONE

The Magic Leaf

The first thing you have to know about homeopathy is that it is a form of medicine. Which is to say that it is clumsy. Unwieldy. That it functions within a particular viewpoint and is manipulated within a type of logic. Like any other medicine, it is ever evolving. It is both science and art and involves both a practice and a philosophy—all of which may be said to be healing in nature.

Like any other form of medicine, sometimes it works, sometimes it doesn't. Sometimes a perfect boob will come up with the right remedy and give it and miracles will result. Other times a genius practitioner will miss the obvious need for Sulphur and give instead a handful of other remedies, all of which fizzle and fail.

The best way to sum it up is to bastardize the words of Abraham Lincoln: homeopathy works for some of the people all of the time, all of the people some of the time, but it won't work for all of the people all of the time.

Again, this is because it is a form of medicine.

And it probably is best, in considering the pluses and minuses of homeopathy, to start by dealing with what makes a medicine a medicine.

What Is Medicine?

That seems an odd question in today's world I know, largely because we were born into a culture that is filled with medicines. Crammed with medicines. They are everywhere. They line the aisles in stores and are photographed like movie stars in our magazines. They come in nice packages with bright colors and the pills look like candy and the liquids look like soda and they have such sweet, loving names. And it has only gotten worse since our government has relaxed its controls on the pharmaceutical industry and our television screens are now filled with dapple-dawn images of happy people swinging in swings over grassy lawns, so happy and so free because they took their purple pills.

We have to take the time to look a bit deeper and come to see that these colors and tastes have nothing to do with medicine and with what makes medicine "medicinal." Medicine has to do with healing, not with selling. Medicine may come sealed in plastic or it may come wrapped in dirty burlap. The packaging and the medicine's healing virtue have as much to do with each other as do the proverbial book and its cover.

No, what makes a medicine a medicine is its ability to create a *change* of some sort in the living body. And that's pretty much it.

> . . . what makes a medicine a medicine is its ability to create a *change* of some sort in the living body.

All modern medicine comes from the wellspring of ancient medicine. It all comes from the herbal pharmacies of the ancient world. And how could it not? We are living on the same planet and we have the same natural resources with which to feed ourselves and protect ourselves. We are breathing the same air and drinking the same water, as did the ancients. In the same way, we are healing ourselves in the same manner that the ancients did. The fact that our pills are now purple and many of our medicines are made from chemical compounds based on ancient herbs or minerals does not change the fact that, refined or not, things just have not changed that much over the years.

The Birth of Medicine

Think about it. The birth of medicine involved a shift that was, at once simple and profound. Some ancient family had a child they loved and that child got sick. There may or may not have been a name for that sickness in their language, but their beloved child was not eating, perhaps she was vomiting, shaking, and getting weaker and weaker. That child was very sick. Up until a certain unknown and unknowable moment in human history, all that that family could do was cry, hold the baby tight, keep the baby warm, and hope for the best. If they had a belief of a deity, they would also pray.

Then one day, someone tried putting a leaf from a certain bush on the baby's head and the baby felt better. Or they gave the baby water from a certain spring and the baby got better.

Think of the implications of that moment. Your baby is sick one day, and resting and happily gurgling the next day. And it was all because of you. Because you did something, you used some tool and that action was effective. Your baby lived because of you.

That moment had to create a powerful cultural shift. That ancient family must have called over the neighbors to look at the baby, to hear the story of their victory.

And more important, that moment of healing had to shift how they saw their world. Suddenly, it had to occur to them that they did not simply have to sit around and live their lives hoping for the best. They could not just fear disease, but they could battle against it and conquer it.

Think how valuable the leaves of that bush would suddenly become. The day before they may have been something that were used only for shade or to feed the animals. Now they were something powerful, something magical.

That couldn't have helped but send that family out into the world around them. From that time forward, they must have not only protected their magical plant but also have gone in search of others. After all, if this bush was magical, who's to say that another one is not even more powerful. Or perhaps that rock was better still. Or the blood of this bird the most magical thing of all. So, in "inventing" medicine, that ancient family had to have sent their community further into the world and profoundly changed the way they lived their lives as they became active where once they were passive.

They began a search for new and improved medicines that continues today.

Sometimes they were on to something real. Sometimes they could use the leaf again, and again another baby with the same sort of illness would get well. After seeing it work again and again, they would know what that leaf could do. But sometimes experience would show them that they were just lucky when they used that first leaf. The baby was getting well, all on his own. When they tried that same leaf again, under the same circumstances, nothing would happen. Then they would have to try something else.

It was all trial and error.

And it remains trial and error today. No matter how much more sophisticated the medical trials, and how much more dynamic the errors, when we learn that a common medication does indeed relieve your arthritis pain but at the same time causes a heart attack, nothing really has changed. We are fools to believe that modern medicine has made changes in the fundamentals of health and healing. We are, after all, still growing old and dying. With or without tubes, noisy machines and medicine, we will still someday leave this Earth behind.

What Makes Medicine *Medicinal*?

Okay, back to what makes medicine medicinal.

First you have to have something that creates a change. That change may be small or it may be profound. That gives the medicine its relative power, its *virtue*.

And that change may be for the better or for the worse. After all, it is the circumstances at hand that largely determine what is "better" or "worse" in the case of a particular disease. The person who has diarrhea will think that the medicine that would help the person with constipation is a rather terrible thing. But that person with three days of constipation will welcome it.

So a medicine used under the wrong circumstances may be said to be a poison. This is
why our first homeopaths commented that "the
stronger the poison, the stronger the cure." In
other words, the more violent the change the
substance creates, the more powerful it may
be as a healing tool. If used under the correct
circumstances, if used in the correct way.

> The more violent the change
> a substance creates, the
> more powerful it may be as
> a healing tool. If used under
> the correct circumstances,
> if used in the correct way.

It also has to be used in a safe way. And given the fact that substances like arsenic
were part of the common medicines a few hundred years ago, it is safe to say that a
large part of our medical trial and error has been to find a medicine that was strong
enough to be effective, yet benign enough to leave the patient alive after you have
cured him.

In today's practice of medicine we have sort of divided up the responsibility for
selecting the circumstances that dictate the use of a given medicine and the responsibility for seeing to it that only safe medicines are used at all. In the past, it was the
responsibility of the individual practitioner both to find a medicine and then to test it
for safety and reliability. Today, our government attempts—and all too often fails—to
identify which medicines are safe to use and which are not. We also pretend that the
pharmaceutical firms assist the government in making sure that everything in our
medicine chests are safe, despite ongoing proof to the contrary.

Therefore, it is the responsibility of the government and industry jointly to create
a culture of safe medicine and it is then left to the individual practitioner to choose
wisely among these many supposedly safe and effective medicines and to use them as
healing tools.

The role of the medicine practitioner is to identify the patient's circumstances
correctly—to play a very good round of "Name that Disease" and to correctly decide
just what is going on that this patient became sick to begin with. And because our
map of treatment—which is to say our choice or of medicine or medicines which will
be effective in combating that particular ailment—is dependent upon the practitioner naming the correct disease, this particular role is key. If, for instance, that practitioner thinks a case of acute kidney failure is simply a case of the flu, he then is very
likely to use his medicines incorrectly and to poison when he means to cure. This is
the dangerous flaw in our medical thinking—we assume we can control diseases simply by naming and grouping their symptoms. This leads to an even more dangerous
flaw—letting the name of that disease create a map for treatment from which we
never deviate until it is too late. These are deep and fatal flaws in the way we practice
medicine and they are flaws that must be corrected.

When we gather symptoms into groups and name them, and then decide that no matter who that patient is and how they are experiencing this particular bout of that disease that the same medicine or group of medicines will always be of value, is to behave like that caveman who laid the leaf from a particular tree on his sick baby's head. We need to go deeper in our understanding of healing. We deserve a better form of medicine and a better system of healing.

In an attempt to fix this flaw, modern medicine has put a great deal of time and energy into developing tests. A simple blood test can now tell us whether we are dealing with flu or kidney failure. The problem with that method of practice is twofold. First, it has created a system of medicine that is ever more top-heavy and impersonal. Because of the cost of these tests and because of the dangerous whims of insurance companies, who often dictate who gets what test and when, many patients are now finding themselves with less and less real medical care that can make the difference in a serious situation. We have let money and the profit motive of the insurance companies dictate who can now afford to have medical care.

Second, and perhaps even more serious, our dependence on medical testing has created an entire generation of practitioners of all sorts—and, remember, I am not yet differentiating between homeopaths and allopaths here—who can no more identify a disease than a modern eighth grader can now do square roots without a calculator.

This is not to say that medical testing and technology are not valuable tools for the wise practitioner to use in the practice of medicine, but that the wise practitioner *knows* that they are only tools. They cannot replace the practitioner in his compassion and his understanding of his patient as a human being.

We have drained the humanity and, yes, the *magic* out of medicine and replaced it with money and we are now paying a terrible price.

CHAPTER TWO

Prince Charming's Kiss

Since we have to begin at the beginning, we not only have to identify just what medicine is, we also have to consider symptoms and what they are as well. But even before we can do that, we have to define just what a patient is. See, for many practitioners of both allopathic and homeopathic medicine, the patient and his symptoms are, sadly, rather interchangeable. And they all too often put their efforts into treating the damn symptoms instead of the patient *with* symptoms. And while this distinction may seem to be slight, the differences in the result of treatment are profound.

What Is a Patient?

It's sad really that this question actually had to be dealt with, but modern medicine, which is to say *allopathic* medicine, has created a profound change in the idea of exactly who and what we treat when we give medical treatment.

So the fundamental question remains, exactly what are we treating when we give medical treatment? Are we treating a disease, which is to say, a group of symptoms common to everyone who has been given the same disease diagnosis? Or are we treating a person who happens to have a group of symptoms common to everyone who has been given the same disease diagnosis? The answer to this single question to a large extent defines and dictates whether the patient receives allopathic or homeopathic treatment.

For the allopath, the treatment is used to combat a particular disease, with the belief that, once that disease is blocked, suppressed, or eliminated—whichever is possible to a given disease state—then good health must result.

For the homeopath, the treatment must always be given to the patient himself or herself. And that patient is seen as a fully rounded being—body, mind, and spirit—in whom there exists a wide range of symptoms, good and bad and indifferent. Whether a symptom is considered to be good or bad is largely determined by the patient himself or herself, by whether or not they perceive a given symptom or group of symptoms as in some way limiting or undermining their quality of life. Symptoms that neither limit the patient nor cause him discomfort are at least benign. Others may be actually considered evidence of a state of good health in that they actually contribute to the patient's ability to live life well and in a state of freedom, as we shall see.

The homeopath would not agree with the allopath that an innate state of good health underlies the presence of a disease and that one need only to remove the disease state that has somehow attacked the innocent patient (watch and note how often allopaths put the medical journey toward health in military terms, with germs "attacking" and "wars" on given disease), and the patient will be immediately returned to a state of good health that was imprisoned somewhere within him all along.

This is a sort of fairy tale approach to health and healing, in which the disease is like some sort of curse placed upon the innocent patient. They have eaten a poison apple and fallen under its spell. The medicine then becomes Prince Charming's kiss, which removes the curse and restores the patient.

The homeopath, on the other hand, sees each person's health state as part of the complex blend that makes them the unique being that they are. When they approach treating a patient with any sort of disease—acute or chronic—that disease state has to be first seen as a state of change, a movement in that patient's particular blend of symptoms that has moved them toward illness, which is to say toward a state of weakness or limitation or pain. This, of course, suggests that perhaps homeopaths see symptoms, since they can be good or bad, as things that are always there, that cannot be removed by medical treatment. And this is indeed the way homeopaths see symptoms.

> This is a fairy-tale approach to health and healing, in which the disease is like some curse placed upon the innocent patient. They have eaten a poison apple and fallen under its spell. The medicine then becomes Prince Charming's kiss, which removes the curse and restores the patient.

Diseases, like everything else, are part of the patients' lives. They are manifestations of the particular patient's life force, as it has been stressed by life, the environment, and any number of other forces, including the allopathic boogeymen—viruses and bacteria. In fact, diseases and symptoms can be seen as a sign of good health at some level, since those patients whose life forces have become totally depleted may actually become too weak and too ill for their bodies to manifest symptoms. They may be too sick to get sick.

So, in the homeopathic world view, here we have the patient, a whole person, a being who innately—given his genetic makeup, his lifestyle, his diet, his age, and so on—tends toward a particular state of health. And now something has created a change. That something can be again lifestyle related or it could be caused by a mechanical injury or a virus—on a profound level it doesn't really matter the actual cause, as the homeopathic treatment for an allergy or a common cold will at least start out the same as long as the symptoms experienced will be the same. But the change has happened and the patient's symptoms have shifted toward the negative. It is then the homeopath's role to help identify the change and to work with the symptoms in such a way that the patient's ability to overcome the symptoms is enhanced and the patient moves toward a state of improved health.

More on this later, that is, on the goals of treatment and how they relate to acute, chronic and even deeper illnesses. But try and understand this now: the homeopath does not believe that a state of good health necessarily underlies the disease state. It is the goal of the homeopath's treatment that the patient be left, after homeopathic treatment, in at least as healthy a state as he was in before the onset of the illness. And even more often, it is the homeopath's goal that the patient be left in a state of permanently improved health.

To conclude this section, it must be remembered that the patient is always the target of the homeopath's treatment. The patient is always seen as a unique and whole being, one who will respond to a given treatment in a unique manner. The homeopath, therefore, cannot ever allow himself to assume anything. There never can be a homeopathic medicine that can be said to be "good for" a particular disease. Homeopathic medicines can only be measured in their actions to the greatest degree of particularity in the greatest number of possible cases tracked. And the actions of these remedies can then be matched to the greatest degree of particularity possible to the symptoms—good and bad and indifferent—that the patient is experiencing in order to bring about a match between the patient and the medicine. This is how homeopathic remedies are appropriately selected and used. This is how homeopathic healing takes place.

And this is one way in which homeopathic treatment is separate from, and indeed in opposition to, allopathic treatment. This has always been and will always be the case. There are no homeopathic medicines available for particular diseases. So there are no easy answers. You cannot, as a homeopath, allow yourself to see the disease as suggesting a particular remedy or group of remedies as the solution. No, with each new case, with each new patient, even the patient who is presenting the symptoms of a disease that you've seen a million times before, you still have to start at the beginning and work through the process. You still have to do the work required for homeopathic healing to take place.

The homeopath is always aware that he himself is no Prince Charming and he has no magic kiss to offer to overcome the apple's poison.

What Are Symptoms?

So, just as the allopath and the homeopath disagree as to what the target of their treatment is, they also disagree on as fundamental a definition as the word *symptom*.

As I have already said, the allopath connotes symptoms with illness. The homeopath, on the other hand, sees symptoms as a fundamental sign of life, as a fundamental sign that the life force within the patient is functioning to the point that that being is still reacting to their environment.

> The homeopath is always aware that he himself is no Prince Charming and he has no magic kiss to offer to overcome the apple's poison.

Symptoms, therefore, may be considered to be reactions—the body's reaction to the presence of something toxic (as with the common cold, in which the body seeks to flush the invading virus from the system), or an overreaction to something that in all reality is quite benign. (And what is an allergy but the immune system going into overdrive and identifying something as benign as dust or dog hair or peanuts and targeting the presence of these things as reason enough to react, react, react?)

Everything in life, it may be said, is a matter of action and reaction. Every argument with a loved one, every physical illness, every physical aspect of life is a matter of push me, pull you. We learned it in elementary science—for every action, there is an equal and opposite reaction. With that basic concept we were given pretty much all the information we need to know to live fruitful, happy, and healthy lives.

I'll get into how that plays into medicine in a moment, but let's stay a bit longer on symptoms.

Allopaths confuse symptoms with diseases. The symptoms of disease are not the disease itself, but are, rather, your body's reaction to the presence of what may be called the "disease agent." Something has become part of your being and it has been identified, rightly or wrongly, as reason enough for your immune system to start to react.

And sometimes your immune system is quite right to react, to begin to try to burn the invader with fever, or to flush it away with mucus, or purge it altogether with vomiting. But sometimes it is wrong as well. Sometimes the immune system can be as nervous as Barney Fife with a loaded pistol. Sometimes it reacts when there is, in all reality, nothing whatsoever wrong. Just as we sometimes can be right when we suspect that a friend said something bad about us behind our backs, we can, just as often, be quite wrong and they never for a moment spoke against us.

Medical doctors used to have a word for it; they called it the "wisdom of the body." And that sounds good, but, in all actuality, our bodies are no more innately wise than are our brains. In truth, our bodies, our immune systems, have to live and learn just like the rest of us have to. Our bodies have to face an ongoing onslaught of invaders, toxins, and just plain new catalysts of all sorts in order for that body, in time, to be able to better differentiate between the threats and the innocent bystanders.

It is therefore a key component of any form of medicine, allopathic or homeopathic, that the practitioners thereof learn and learn well how to identify the symptoms that will best allow them to form an opinion as to the best path toward health for the individual patient.

To do this, the practitioner has to have the ability to understand that patient. They have to have some idea of that patient's "normal" level of health—what he or she feels like when they feel that they are healthy. Some of us, after all, have been gifted with a wonderful, healthy body. But others, even when they are as healthy as they can be, always seem to have something or other wrong with them.

Whatever that patient's normal state of health may be, it has to be understood if the practitioner is to then understand what has changed in that status quo so that the patient now is feeling ill. Therefore, it is the change that is most important. The physician must come to understand exactly what has changed in the patient if they have any hope in reversing or in any other way shaping that change. And the practitioner must also have some understanding as to the circumstances surrounding that change. As any good allergist would ask, the practitioner must ask what has changed in the patient's environment—what did they eat, touch, smell or in any other physical manner contact that might have caused the reactive state of disease. Further, the practitioner must try to gather the timetable of the event. Has this disease been building for weeks or months or even years, or did the change come quickly, in a matter of hours?

I think that any good medical professional, allopathic or homeopathic, will get this far. All will seek to gather information as to what exactly is bothering the patient, asking for more or less detail about each symptom, and trying to piece this information on a timetable of sorts. But here is what makes the difference—the allopath stops here. The timetable of symptoms is then labeled with a name—a disease diagnosis. And, based on that diagnosis, the course of appropriate treatment is set in place. This course of treatment involves not only the use of a limited set of drugs that are considered to be effective for that disease, but also perhaps a change in diet, or in exercise, or in climate (environment).

The homeopath never makes that simplistic leap to a disease diagnosis. In fact, classic homeopaths will often avoid giving a name to a set of symptoms, both because they themselves do not want to be influenced by that name and fall prey to the idea that you can treat a disease with a specific drug or drugs, and because they do not want to put the full weight of that diagnosis—that dreadful word like "cancer" or "AIDS"— on the already depleted patient. This is not to say that a homeopath will in any way hide any information from a patient and will not tell them whatever they need or want to know, but it is important to state that the homeopath will never stop there, will never surrender their skill and art to a word that only creates fear and dread and that, in a very real way, is meaningless.

If, like a homeopath, you refuse to accept that the name of the disease implies the plan of action for its defeat, then that disease name becomes a meaningless thing. And, depending on the fear that a particular disease name inspires, the stamping of a patient's condition with a name may actually harm the patient. The patient can become a good deal weaker and less likely to recover once they have been given their disease diagnosis. Once the terrifying word has been spoken and, in the speaking, has confirmed their deepest fears.

The homeopath in the same situation will simply stay with the symptoms. They will emphasize their own ability to understand the change that has taken place from a state in which that particular patient felt healthy to one in which they feel that they are ill. The homeopath will try to understand how the onset of illness has transformed the patient on every level of being. They will therefore not be satisfied just to know the full range of physical symptoms, but will also wish to understand how the illness has affected the patient mentally. Are they thinking as clearly as usual, or do they feel foggy or disconnected in their illness? And emotionally, does the patient feel afraid in their illness, or angry, or any other strong emotion?

Even after working to understand this, the homeopath will stay with the symptoms. They will not abandon them and make the leap to giving a single name to the whole cluster of symptoms and then basing a treatment on that name. No, they will work to understand the patient as they are at this moment, and then try to understand what they were like when healthy. And they will try to understand the change that has occurred in all of its ramifications. Only then will they be ready to treat.

When the homeopath treats, he will do so based on what is called the "drug diagnosis." This is, for the homeopath, far more important than the disease diagnosis. In the drug diagnosis, the homeopath will seek to match the total action of a given remedy in all that it is capable of doing for a patient, in terms of physical, mental, and emotional symptoms, with all that the patient is already experiencing in his mind, emotions, and body. If the homeopath is able to match the two—the drug action and the disease state as experienced by this particular patient—then a cure will result.

Don't you see, the fatal flaw in the allopath's art is that he comes to believe that the same drug will have the same action for every patient suffering from the same disease?

The homeopath knows that each of us is unique. Unique in our experience of health and just what constitutes a fully embodied quality of health, and in just what constitutes illness. Each of us is unique in the way we experience even a common cold, some with a sore throat, others with watery eyes. Some with fevers, some with-out; some well again in a day or two, and others in bed sick for a week or more. In truth, we may all be the same species, but we have more things about us that are truly unique than we have things in common. We each have a unique way of being born. I was a breech birth and weeks overdue when labor was finally induced. Others pop out right at nine months with full heads of hair. We each have a unique way of dying and of facing death. And, in between, we each of us have a totally unique way of liv-ing. We may all have immune systems, but no two of them function in exactly the same way.

Stupid, Stupid Allopaths

Much as I have tried over the years to come to accept that those who practice allo-pathic medicine are simply doing the best that they can, I cannot get past the simple point that allopaths just keep making the same two mistakes over and over again.

First, they keep insisting that every patient with the same disease will benefit from the same treatment. And, in insisting on this, they continue to make elderly patients faint and break their hips because their hypertension medicine is too strong, and they open the door for pharmaceutical companies to sell drugs that relieve pain but cause heart attacks. (Am I alone in thinking that this is not an acceptable trade-off and that any warning label short of a skull and crossbones is simply not strong enough?) This first mistake is all too often fatal for the patient. And then the grieving family is told, "We did all that we could." And indeed they did do all that they possi-bly could—they killed the patient.

The second mistake is just as bad. Allopaths insist somehow that they can con-trol the actions of their medications. That they can predict precisely what that drug will do in that patient's body. (The aforementioned pharmaceutical issues should alone give lie to this issue.)

When I defined the word medicine for you, I gave it a very general definition as something that causes a change to take place. That magic leaf.

Now the lifetime that each of us has spent being given every sort of medication, from over the counter candy-coated pills to prescriptions issued just for us, should have taught us something: no medication only does one thing. They all do a whole lot of things in addition to the thing that they were prescribed for in the first place. Cold medicines cause our blood pressure to rise, which can be a critically bad thing if you happen to have high blood pressure in the first place.

And doctors of all sorts are aware of this fact. Every medicine causes a range of changes in the human system. Some create more dramatic or wide-ranging changes than do others. But doctors caught on pretty early on that they really couldn't make a career out of saying, "Well, let's try this pill and see if it helps you or if it turns your skin purple." So they have developed a whole rather top-heavy system in order to deal with the issue.

First, they gave these other changes (other than the one that they actually want the medicine to cause) a name. They call them "side effects." And then, as they always tend to do, they began to list them and record them. Not in order to control them, or to make their medicines safer, no, they record them for the same reason that they name their diseases. Because they operate under some state of wishful thinking in which in naming something they can actually control it. But they cannot.

Look at a *Physician's Desk Reference*. Look up any drug. You will find a paragraph that tells you what the drug is for. Then you will find two, three, or four pages telling you what the side effects are.

Somehow, in making their lists, the allopaths actually seem to think that they can separate out the "primary action" of a drug from its side effects. They seem to sort of anthropomorphize the drug, so that it will, now that everything has been listed for it, cooperate and only work from its primary action and stop doing all the rest of that stuff it used to do.

No, in reality, you cannot sweep side effects aside any more than you can ignore the man behind the curtain once you have seen him.

Each action that a drug pushes onto the patient's being is of equal import, as each action will create an equal and opposite reaction from that patient's being. The body doesn't know which action was primary, and which were side effects. It only knows that changes are being artificially created by the use of a drug and that it now has to deal with those changes as best it can.

Disease and "Artificial Disease"

And some patient's bodies will deal with the "artificial disease" created by the use of the drug better than others.

As an aside, it is important that you begin to think of all drugs—allopathic and homeopathic—as forms of artificial disease. If, after all, a disease state is nothing more than a cluster of uncomfortable reactions in our body—reactions to things that we have tasted, smelled, or touched, and so on—then drugs, which cause all sorts of changes in our bodies, minds, and emotions, really are artificial diseases of a sort.

And all that homeopaths and allopaths are really trying to do in giving you medicine is to set up an artificial disease state that will in some way bring you back to a state of health.

It is the manner in which this artificial disease state is created and the thinking behind it that determines whether a treatment is allopathic or homeopathic. It all comes down to how you deal with the symptoms.

And treating symptoms is what the next chapter is all about.

CHAPTER THREE

Equal and Opposite

It is very simple really. When you are faced with a patient complaining of disease symptoms, there are really only a limited number of things you can do. You can work against those symptoms and try to beat them back. Or you can work with those symptoms and try to bring them forth. Or you can do nothing and hope that the patient is strong enough to withstand those symptoms and, ultimately, just get well on his own.

Most books on homeopathy will tell you that the allopath makes the first choice and works against the symptoms and tries to beat them back, or suppress them. And this is certainly true.

But I believe that, in many cases, the allopathic doctor actually makes the third choice and does little or nothing of real medical value. Ultimately, the allopath does nothing and hopes that you get well on your own.

On the face of it, allopathic medicine is all about working against symptoms, struggling against disease. As I have said before, allopathic thought is equal to military thought. The disease is an invader that can somehow be separated from the patient. It is as if a tick had attached itself to a leg and has only to be pulled free for the whole situation to be fixed.

So the patient's invading symptoms are noted and listed. And a diagnosis is made. And based on that diagnosis, a medicine is given whose action it is to work in direct opposition to the disease state itself. So, the patient with a runny nose will be given a medicine whose perceived action it is to dry up noses in the vast majority of cases. The whole idea here is not to strengthen the patient's system, allowing the patient to throw off the disease, but, instead, to simply interfere with the patient's experience of the disease. As the television ads tell us, you can take this pill and your nose will dry up for a whole eight hours (more or less, or to a lesser or greater degree, sometimes safely and sometimes not so safely, depending upon the individual patient's reaction to the medication).

The fact that the medication, even when it works well, is only a Band-Aid that lets you pretend for a brief period of time that you do not have the disease that you actually *do* have (so that you can go back to work earlier and spread the virus to everyone whose hand you shake and who breathes the same air as you in the elevator) is bad enough. But there is a deeper issue, and that is the fact that while this sort of approach to healing is at best useless, at worst, it can actually damage the patient and weaken their overall health.

Working against symptoms is essentially a waiting game. You are, in giving medicine to set up an artificial disease state to counter the natural state at hand, attempting to buy the patient time with your treatment, nothing more. You are trying to buy them the time for their own system to heal itself.

So, the much-touted allopathic medicine, in all reality is doing nothing of real value.

Think about it. Does a painkiller stop a headache, or cause it to end sooner? No, it simply masks the pain. Does it ever strengthen your system so that the likelihood of the next headache becomes lessened? Certainly not. All that painkiller does is simply interfere with your ability to sense the pain that you are actually in. And since it can be assumed that a headache in most cases is a self-limiting or acute condition, it can also be assumed that, if we can block your experience of your headache pain, by the time the painkiller's effects wear off your headache will have gone away on its own.

So what is really accomplished when you take a painkiller for a headache or arthritis or back pain, or any other form of pain other than a brief ability to block the symptoms that you are really feeling? Don't we deserve something more from our dominant system of medicine? Don't we deserve a system that doesn't just give up on the idea of pain and where it is coming from and what it means? Something better than a system that simply gives your pain a name—"headache" or "arthritis"—and then gives you a pill to relieve that pain for a short time.

And, listen, I know something about pain. I used to have migraines so bad that sometimes I would be in bed in a dark room for more than a day at a time. When I felt that first twinge in my forehead that I came to recognize as the onset of the pain, I knew that soon I would be able to bear no light, no sound, and certainly no food. I remember days of literally crying in pain.

I took the painkillers and I was happy to get them. But, even though I felt the blessed relief of pain with the first pill, I knew that this wouldn't stop the next headache or the next. Every time a thunderstorm approached, I would feel the change in the barometer and I would feel the headache coming. As a storm approached, my life was put on hold. Appointments were cancelled. If I were in car, I turned that car around and headed home.

But after what seemed a lifetime of this, I knew that there had to be a way in which I could bring about a more fundamental change in my life, one that would go beyond the actions of the painkillers and would literally set me free from this pain once and for all.

Thankfully, I found it. And once I was healed of these migraines, I was totally and completely healed. I haven't had one for twenty years. I now sometimes get headaches like other people do. They are little things, gone in an hour or two all on their own.

I do know about pain. I know all about pain that is so severe that you would make any deal, swallow any pill to make it go away. But I had to reach the point at which I felt I deserved a better sort of treatment, a deeper treatment—that I deserved to be free of the pain once and for all.

So I can only conclude that, if you are suffering pain, or if someone you love is suffering pain, that you have the right to expect more from your medicine. You have the right to a healing that is, as Samuel Hahnemann said, rapid, gentle, and permanent.

> . . . you have the right to expect more from your medicine. You have the right to a healing that is, as Samuel Hahnemann said, rapid, gentle, and permanent.

Suppression

There is, unfortunately, an even greater downside to the allopathic approach to medicine.

Again, think about it, think about how the continued use of allopathic medicine makes you feel, and how well it works in multiple doses. Does allopathic medicine continue to work as well the second, third, or fourth time as it did the first? Does that painkiller work as well each time if you are not one of those who gets just one headache a year, but are instead one of the unfortunates who gets migraine after migraine after migraine?

The same is true of insomnia. The sleeping pill that works so well the first night will not continue to work as well night after night after night. In time you will need a stronger and stronger dose to recreate the original effect. And this is because all the drug was doing in the first place was suppressing symptoms, and suppressing symptoms always comes at a price.

The truth is that when you suppress the symptom, when you push it aside to separate the patient from his experience of actual pain, you, in time, will actually weaken the patient in terms of his illness, making that illness stronger and that patient weaker. That patient who takes more and more pills to fall asleep will, in time, not only still not be sleeping, but will find no relief from those pills at all, no matter how many they take. Further, the pills will become toxic to their system. The fact our treatment centers are literally filled with patients who have become addicted to the painkillers that were originally medically prescribed for them stands as testament of their toxicity.

Just as we cannot heal ourselves emotionally by pretending that we do not have anger and hatred against a father who abused us—in order to get well at some point or other we actually have to admit the abuse and deal with it directly—in the same way we cannot heal physically if we continue to put all our energy into suppressing the disease symptoms that are themselves warnings of changes within our bodies, changes that may present a challenge to life itself.

At some point we have to get beyond our love of the short-term solution of pain relief and go deeper. In our culture we seem to always be willing to choose the short-term solution over the long-term result. And this is how it is played out in terms of our health. We are willing to sell out our long-term health and strength so that we can take this pill in front of us and get through the headache that we have today. Tomorrow's headache, we figure, will take care of itself. After all, aren't there a virtually infinite number of pills available for the next headache and the next and the next? And aren't those pills readily available and aggressively marketed, making for a multi-billion dollar industry that is built around the idea of deadening pain?

Before I go on, let me note that I am in no way opposed to the prudent use of painkillers. There are times and circumstances in which they are a blessing. In the same way, I am not universally against the use of antibiotics. In some circumstances, they can be true lifesavers. The same may be said for any number of modern allopathic medications, when used prudently.

Let's face it, the allopathic medical industry is just filled with eager beavers. They are always busy, always finding new medicines or new uses for old medicines. (And when they get their hands on a medicine, they tend to act like pit bulls with bones. Nothing makes them let go. Remember a few years ago when researchers found new and supposedly safe uses of thalidomide? Wouldn't you think that the hundreds of children who were born without arms after the drug was given to their pregnant mothers would be reason enough for someone to say, "Let's just let this one go." But no, some researchers just had to ask the question, "But what if they *weren't* pregnant?")

The problem with their zeal is that, as they develop newer and stronger medicines—and I have always wondered why, if the medicines worked to begin with, they needed to be, as the commercials tell us, "new and improved"—they are developing them from the same wrongheaded notions that have been in place since the allopathic era began two thousand years ago.

The fact that these drugs are "new and improved" only makes them all the more suppressive and, therefore, all the more dangerous.

And, while I'm off topic for a second, let me note that I find myself both in awe of and extremely interested in the fledgling science of genetic medicine, as it may well represent the first actual change in the nature of medicine in the history of mankind. It may well prove in time to be a third type of medicine, one that is neither allopathic nor homeopathic.

But until the development of a truly new form of medicine, I cannot help but note that the allopathic system that we have in place in our culture is greatly in need of change. I cannot help but speak out against building an entire system on the use of medicines that by both their nature and use are ultimately useless at best and, at worst, quite toxic.

Working *with* Symptoms

Having exhausted two of the three possible approaches to symptoms associated with disease, there remains only one more possible approach: working with the symptoms.

But what, exactly, does this mean?

Ridiculous as it sounds, it means that we are going to try doing exactly that—we are going to actually enhance the symptoms. Instead of telling that runny nose that it is time for it to dry up, we are going to give it full permission to run as much as it can.

In action, this means that we are going to give the person with a runny nose a medicine that, if it were given to a perfectly healthy person would give that person a runny nose. This idea, that "like cures like" is the very heart of homeopathy. It was the concept with which Samuel Hahnemann (1755–1843) began the quiet revolution in healthcare that has now stood the test of two centuries of practice.

When you first hear this idea, it sounds pretty silly. It even sounded a bit crazy to Hahnemann himself, I am sure. He had come upon the notion because of a specific herbal remedy; one that related to the European expansion into the New World. You see, European explorers had, upon reaching the shores of South America, fallen prey to a particularly potent fever. And that the natives had shown the white men that by chewing a particular bark they could overcome the fever. Now, there was nothing particularly amazing about that, it was just another form of herbal medicine, another magic leaf.

The Jesuit missionaries brought some of the bark back with them to Europe. And Hahnemann, in exploring his developing theories of the nature of medicine, himself ingested the bark, although he himself was in a state of good health. Hahnemann found that, as he chewed the bark, he began to experience the symptoms that were commonly linked to the fever state itself. In time, these symptoms faded, but this experience was something that stayed with Hahnemann. Something, no doubt, he had to mull over a great deal. But in the end something became very clear: that the chinchona bark only had the power to cure the fever because it also had the power to cause the fever.

This was the birth of a new concept, one that held that the power of any given medicine lay in that medicine's ability to create a state of "artificial disease."

What Hahnemann also understood was that, in order to make full and proper use of a medicine, a practitioner had to understand and make use of not just the primary or most hoped for action of the remedy, but the myriad actions of the remedy—its entire sphere of activity in the patient's body, mind, and emotions. Therefore, the chinchona bark, because it had the medicinal action of creating a fever in a healthy person, would also have the action of removing a fever in the patient who already had a fever. But it could only cure the fever that was similar in all of its symptoms to the symptoms that chinchona could create. In other words, if the chinchona fever was one in which the patient was chilled to the bone while in the fever state and one in which the patient was thirsty and terribly fearful and agitated, then the medicine could not be very helpful in the case of a fever in which the patient was hot and sweaty, not thirsty or resting quietly. The entirety of the patient's symptoms had to match as closely as possible the entirety of the artificial disease state that the medicine could create. Then cure was the result.

In one quick insight, Hahnemann made the case as to why allopathic medicines just don't do the job. First, they are selected by virtue of the disease diagnosis—which is to say that, in terms of allopathic treatment, fever one is fever two is fever three. And second, allopathic drugs would not, if given to a healthy person, necessarily create an artificial disease that would mimic the one that was naturally occurring. They would, in fact, create an artificial disease state that was quite the opposite of the one that was naturally occurring. So cure was quite impossible by this method.

Now, what Hahnemann lacked two hundred years ago was a simple explanation as to why this was the case. Today, we have a commonly known and easily understood law of physics that explains why medicine works the way it does—both allopathic and homeopathic medicine. I've touched on it earlier, but let's consider it again.

Newton's third law of motion states that "for every action there is an equal and opposite reaction." Is there anyone who does not understand this very simple premise, or who would argue that it is not true?

We just have not yet applied it to medicine. But give it a try.

If you have a patient who cannot sleep and you give him an allopathic medicine that puts him to sleep, you will get an excellent result the first night. That is because the patient will be sucker-punched by the drug's action. His system is unaware of what it has been given. And it has no strategy in place as to just what to do about this particular catalyst.

But, if you have a patient who was not just having a particularly stressful day when they could not sleep, but often finds himself or herself sleepless for weeks at a time, you will find, if he takes these pills often enough, that very soon the pills just are not working very well. This is because the patient's system is becoming aware of the changes caused by the medicine and is reacting to them. For every action there is an equal and opposite reaction. The first time you give the sleeping pill, you are working off of the primary action of the medicine. And the patient sleeps. But the more you take that insomniac and try to push them toward sleep, the more you will create a reaction within the patient's system—one that actually will make them all the more awake.

The error that the practitioners of allopathic medicine make is to think that a cure will come about through the primary action of the medicine. In order to believe this, they have to believe that all patients react to medicine in the same way, which they do not. They also have to try to pretend that they can separate out the primary action of the medicine from all the side effects, which they cannot. And they have to ignore one of the basic laws of the universe, which tells us that for every action there is an equal and opposite reaction, which means that that primary action of the medicine will always be followed by an equal and opposite reaction which it is quite impossible for them to control.

Homeopathy, on the other hand, works by virtue of what is called the "secondary action," which is nothing more really than the body's reaction to the primary action of the medicine.

It all comes down to "Sez who?" and "Sez me." Because all medicine is a matter of shoving, like kids on the playground. The primary action of any medicine is just like that initial shove on the playground. Then it is a matter of waiting to see what the reaction will be. Allopathy is "Sez who?" medicine, which is to say that it relies upon the initial shove of the medicine to do the work, and then tries to ignore the shove back—the "Sez me" that the body screams when it reacts to the medicine—by calling it a side effect. Homeopathy, on the other hand, is "Sez me" medicine, since the primary action of the remedy is similar in action to the disease state as the patient is already experiencing it. Which is to say that it has the power to create these same symptoms in a well person that are already being experienced by the patient all on his own. The appropriate remedy, however, is also just slightly stronger in impact than is the natural disease state. This causes the secondary action of the medicine—the reactive state, the shove back against that initial shove—to move the patient's system away from the symptoms that they are already experiencing and toward cure.

The homeopath, therefore, takes that insomniac and first places the insomnia as an individual symptom within the context of all the other symptoms that the patient is also experiencing at the same time and then second selects the remedy that seems to best match the patient as a whole being experiencing a full range of symptoms. This will always be the procedure, whether that patient has acute insomnia or has never experienced a full night's sleep in their lifetime.

Say that remedy is Coffea, which is, interestingly enough, taken from coffee. The patient needing this would be an excited insomniac, one who gets worked up at bedtime so that he not only can't sleep but has trouble keeping still. This is a great remedy to remember in cases of toothache as well, when that patient just can't stop jumping around from the pain. It also can help kids who are too excited to sleep on Christmas Eve.

Anyway, the homeopath gives that well-chosen remedy, whose power it is to create in a healthy person not only the insomnia, but also the other symptoms that the patient is experiencing. And then he lets nature take its course.

> For every action there is indeed an equal and opposite reaction. And our inborn healing mechanism works by this principle.

The action of the remedy will stimulate the same symptoms that the patient is already experiencing, and the patient already has insomnia. But then, upon taking the remedy Coffea, the patient will begin his or her equal and opposite reaction to that remedy's action, and his system will rise up against the insomnia, and sleep will result. And, best of all, this sleep is a natural sleep, not a drugged state, not a suppression of symptoms, but an expression of health.

Once this remedy has worked and the patient can sleep, their insomnia is cured. The symptom has been expressed from the patient's being, instead of suppressed deeper into it. So the cure, when it takes place, is permanent.

And perhaps best of all, the cure leaves the patient in a state of health that is as good or better than the one he or she enjoyed before treatment. There is no weakening of the system, no suppression, no side effects. The well-chosen remedy has taken into account the full range of symptoms of the illness and matched them to the full range of actions of the remedy. Cure results, and you're done.

Now, the fact that this works so well—and I have seen it work just as well hundreds of times for hundreds of different diseases over the years—doesn't mean it's easy.

You have to have the knowledge to find the right remedy. And then you have to know how to use that remedy, what potency, what dosage, when to begin treatment, when to stop, when and whether or not you should go on to a second remedy. None of this is particularly easy. And when you are struggling to get it right, you may well think rather wistfully of the allopath who only has to choose among a handful of medicines for a particular disease, where you have to consider thousands of remedies in each case, as there is no way to link a particular remedy to a particular disease.

But the homeopathic method actually works. It actually allows for the possibility that illness can be cured and that patients don't have to take multiple medications day after day for the rest of their lives just to sustain the level of disease that they have come to think of as normal.

I made the choice in my own life a quarter century ago, when I was chronically ill and allopathic medicine abandoned me. I never abandoned it, I never would have. As a sickly child and an even sicker adult, I was the perfect little patient, one who did as he was told, never asked difficult questions, and paid his bills on time.

And what it ultimately got me was the "Nothing more we can do" speech.

Then I needed to find an alternative, and I found one. One that, to my great surprise, actually worked.

This is not to say that homeopathy will always work, or that it is a perfect practice of medicine. No, sometimes it will fail. Sometimes the illness is too great, or the life force is too weak. Sometimes you will, unfortunately, have an idiot for a practitioner.

But Samuel Hahnemann and Isaac Newton were both on to something. For every action there is indeed an equal and opposite reaction. And our inborn healing mechanism works by this principle. Our method of healing is *reactive in nature*. It will react to whatever it suspects is capable of damage, whether that catalyst be environmental in nature, or viral, or medicinal. By working with our symptoms we can resolve—truly resolve—our illnesses and become well.

CHAPTER FOUR

Rapid, Gentle, and Permanent

In the front-piece of this book, I quoted Samuel Hahnemann from his book the *Organon of Medicine*. The particular quote I used came from aphorism #2. I will give you the entire context of that quote in a moment.

Now those who are already students of homeopathy already know that the *Organon* is a slim volume, but within its pages, Hahnemann gave us a complete understanding of the practice of homeopathy. And this information is given in the form of aphorisms, or short quotes.

The first two are, for me, among the most valuable thoughts that Hahnemann ever shared. They are as follows:

- Aphorism #1: "The physician's highest and *only* calling is to make the sick healthy, to cure, as it is called."

- Aphorism #2: "The highest ideal of cure is the rapid, gentle, and permanent restoration of health: that is, the lifting and annihilation of the disease in its entire extent in the shortest, most reliable, and least disadvantageous way, according to clearly realizable principles."

In two short sentences, Hahnemann sets the bar very high indeed for what is acceptable in the practice of medicine and what is appropriate in a patient's level of expectation.

The First Aphorism

In the first aphorism, it is important to note that the italics are Hahnemann's. It is his idea that the physician is to dedicate himself to what was once considered the highest of callings—the restoration of health to those who suffer.

This very short sentence begs that we stop and consider two specific word choices. And since this translation of the *Organon* from the original German is the very best possible, in that this edition of Hahnemann's work, edited by Wenda Brewster O'Reilly, is the finest I have ever seen (more on that and other homeopathic books in Chapter 17), is most scrupulous in word selection, we have to go with the fact that Hahnemann, for reasons of his own, uses the word "physician" and not "doctor" and the word "cure" and not the word "heal." These are vital choices.

First, it is to be hoped that those who dedicate their lives to the healing arts will elect to be physicians and not doctors. If they can manage to do both, so much the better, but the practitioner who is both a doctor and a physician is a rare thing.

The term "doctor" is an earned title. One that takes years of study and struggle to be able to place before one's Christian name. It is, therefore, a sign of education and achievement.

American medicine has for centuries been based in the paternalistic concept that insists, among many other things, that the practitioner be addressed as "Doctor" while the doctor, even one who is a good generation younger than the patient, addresses that patient by his or her first name. To me, this has always been a method by which the doctor's authority is enhanced, whether that particular doctor's level of skill or knowledge is worthy of respect or authority. Those qualities, it seems to me, should be earned through dedication and hard work and not insisted upon by the doctor himself and his beehive of attendants who surround him.

Further, this demand of an honorific title tends to infantilize the patient, in my opinion. The fifty-year-old patient who had to call his thirty-year-old practitioner "Doctor" while that doctor calls him "Henry" is far less likely to ask difficult questions or to demand that the answers to his questions—if he manages to stammer them out—be answered in plain English, instead of the happy jargon that doctors tend to fall back on when they want to put the interview to an end and move the patient out of their office.

Hahnemann, to his credit, while he had been trained as an allopathic doctor before going crazy (at least from the allopath's point of view) and developing the practice of homeopathy, thought that patients deserved something better than doctors. They deserved to be treated by physicians.

And there is quite a bit of difference in the meanings of these words, however often they are mistakenly used interchangeably.

Where the term "doctor" is one that is earned by a specific educational degree and is, in all reality, a legal term, the term "physician" relates to a calling, and not a test score or a state certification. It relates also to a method of practice and an understanding of human nature—to say nothing of the nature of healing—that cannot be taught in a classroom.

Consider the first aphorism again, "The physician's highest and *only* calling is to make the sick healthy, to cure, as it is called." There's that word again, "calling." We've sort of lost the idea of people having callings in our society. For me, it is very telling that about the only people who say that they have felt that they must do the job that they are doing, that they have been "called" to do it are movie stars. They will tell us of the years that they had to go from audition to audition, times when they had to sleep on friends' couches or in cars, all because they knew in their hearts that they were destined to be nominated for an Academy Award.

There was a time in which we heard a great deal about callings. Ministers were called to preach and exhort, teachers were called to raise up a new generation that could inherit this world and make it a better place. And physicians were called for the sole purpose of making the sick healthy, or curing those in weakness or pain.

In that time, I think it was far more common for doctors to be physicians as well. The two ideas—one of an educated and seasoned scientific practitioner and the other of an idealistic and dedicated healer—seemed at one time to more easily be found in one package.

And, let me note that I am making no separation between homeopaths and allopaths in these statements. Nor does Hahnemann. He refers to the physician—not to the homeopath or the allopath. In fact, if you take the time to read the *Organon*, and I hope that you will, you will find that a large portion of the book is not about homeopathy, but, rather, about medicine and about the doctor's search for a cure and the patient's search for healing.

In fact, and this needs to be said—I have far more respect for, and, should I be in need of treatment, I would sooner choose to be treated by an allopath who has studied hard, worked hard, and come to believe wholeheartedly in his particular practice of medicine than I would want to be treated by a half-assed homeopath who was a dabbler in the field of medicine. But face the fact, in our culture, it is far easier for an allopathic physician to be a bit half-assed than it is for a homeopath. A homeopath is an oddity. A homeopath is a bit suspect just by virtue of *being* a homeopath, and so is more likely to be passionately a homeopath than an allopath is likely to be passionately an allopath.

But this is most certainly a generality. I have met half-assed, undereducated, and wooden-headed homeopaths by the dozen. But back to the central issue, and back to Hahnemann's words. According to Hahnemann it is never enough, never acceptable for a practitioner to be half-assed, undereducated, or wooden headed, no matter what type of medicine he or she practices. It is necessary that the person who would be a physician—whose sole function in life it is to "make the sick healthy"—treat their life's work with all due seriousness and to make sure that they fulfill their life's work with skill, dedication, and caring.

But this calling does not, in my opinion, have to necessarily include two aspects usually associated with the position of doctor.

First, I do not believe that a physician ever needs to "make the sick healthy" for money. A calling never needs to translate into a career.

We have lost track in our culture of doing things for the pure love of doing them. All wonderful cooks lay down their pots and pans to try to become Martha Stewart. And, let's face it, if at some point someone with a natural calling toward something does not manage to make money at it, that person's loved ones will make sure that the calling is put aside in the name of earning a living. The world is full of singers and musicians and actors and poets who, because they were not able to make the money that they needed to make from their art, sadly abandoned that art to commerce. In the same way, we have lost all respect for doctors whose offices are not overflowing with eager patients and whose bills are not overpriced beyond all possible reasonable expectation.

We confuse talent with business acumen. And anyone who has had the experience of struggling with a serious disease in recent years has seen the result that this confusion has had on our medical industry.

By all accounts, Samuel Hahnemann had quite a temper. I have been told that he was quite the foot-stamper. So I cannot help but suspect that he might well have put a hole in the floor over our present plight.

The second aspect that contributes to our overall confusion is related to the first. Just as I do not think that a physician needs to be a person who makes a career from his calling, I do not think that a physician needs to be a doctor either. Which is to say, while our government most certainly has the ability to oversee the training of medical professionals and, along with the medical schools, to set certain levels of education and certain proficiency of practice in order to award an individual with the accolade of "doctor," it is my opinion that no governmental body has the ability to grant an individual with the calling that is the fundamental attribute required for a lifetime successfully spent in the practice of medicine.

This is most certainly not to say that I do not think that physicians have to be educated. Quite the opposite. A physician has to have a zeal to learn and understand his medical art that supercedes anything else in his life. And, if that zeal happens to be specifically geared toward allopathic medicine, and if the prospective physician has the funds necessary to get through medical school at a good university, all well and good. But for those who are too poor to get into that fine university, or are the wrong color or religion, or for those whose belief exists outside the realm of allopathic medicine, well, then another form of education may be needed. History is, after all, filled with physicians—herbalists mostly—who were self-taught in their art. My own maternal grandmother was a magnificent herbal healer, she had to be since she was raising eleven children on her own during the Great Depression. She grew the herbs that she needed in her own garden and kept a journal in which she drew pictures of the plants that she used. The journal is, however, useless to us now from a medical point of view, largely because she herself was taught about the use of herbal medicine in her native Italy and often did not know the English name of a given plant. And she most certainly did not know the botanical names for anything. So the journal has no value as a teaching guide. But this little woman managed to get herself and her children safely through the worst economic years this country has ever known and managed to get her children through their childhoods both hale and hearty.

Human medical history is filled with herbalists, tribal healers, and, even, barbers, whose work it was to make the best use possible of the medicinal substances available within the local environment and then pass their knowledge on, either verbally or in the written word, to the next generation, all for the good of the community.

And despite the fact that we now live in a technology-based society that has standardized medical education, can we say that we can be guaranteed proper medical treatment—treatment that is skilled and compassionate—when we walk through the doors of any doctor's office? Of course not. But while I most certainly would never call for the tearing down of our educational or licensing system as they are applied to the practice of medicine, I just can't fully buy into the notion that that system functions as well as we would hope that it would.

The point is that, when it comes to the practice of homeopathy, the whole system pretty much falls apart anyway. After all, it is simply not possible to be a homeopath in the United States. You can be a medical doctor who practices homeopathy, or a naturopathic physician, or, in some places, a nurse practitioner or some other form of medical professional, but you cannot simply be a homeopath.

And it is not really possible to study pure homeopathy within the medical context, either. By this I mean that if you want to study classical homeopathy, you are either going to have to go to some organization or school whose function it is to just teach homeopathy—in which case the diploma you receive after attending that school will have no legal value and will not allow you to actually be a homeopath—or you are going to have to attend a school which offers some legal degree, but which will teach you about things other than homeopathy. Some of these, like naturopathic colleges, will teach homeopathy among many other approaches to medicine, some allopathic and others homeopathic in nature. Others, like traditional medical schools will either ignore homeopathy altogether or will likely equate homeopathy with quackery.

> . . . the best and most knowledgeable homeopaths—those who would fall into the category of physicians—are often lacking the title "doctor." They are often, in fact, self-taught.

So the reality is that, in my experience at least, the best and most knowledgeable homeopaths—those who would fall into the category of physicians—are often lacking the title "doctor." They are often, in fact, self-taught.

Now by no means am I suggesting that you read a few books and then start handing out remedies on a street corner. I am just trying to get across the idea to you that being a doctor is not enough. Not for Hahnemann. No, if you want to "make the sick healthy," you have to be a physician.

The Second Aphorism

The second aphorism is a bitch. Were I a medical student who respected the work of Samuel Hahnemann, it might be enough to persuade me to go into insurance work.

It is very short and simple. "The highest ideal of cure is the rapid, gentle, and permanent restoration of health; that is, the lifting and annihilation of the disease in its entire extent in the shortest, most reliable, and least disadvantageous way, according to clearly realizable principles."

This statement takes no prisoners, although it does exist in the real world. By this I mean that it begins with a bit of an apology when it says, "the highest ideal of cure." This sort of says to me that he was dealing with the healing arts as they should be practiced, and not as they usually are. But to the physician, this aphorism demands that they always try. That their methods be demonstrable in the first place—that they be able to elicit the same response—in other words, that they be able to cure—some large percentage of their patients. And they have to do this in a manner that is "shortest, most reliable, and least disadvantageous."

This brings up the three words that, in my opinion, every patient has the right to expect and every physician has the obligation to try to the best of their skill to provide in terms of cure: rapid, gentle, and permanent.

For the mediocre practitioner, that trio of demands is nearly impossible to achieve. And given my overall belief of the wrong-headedness of allopathy, you can probably guess that I believe that it is all but impossible to achieve these goals through allopathic treatment.

Now, take the three apart, break them down into pairs and you have the sort of medicine that can be achieved by allopaths and homeopaths alike.

Take rapid and permanent for instance. This can be the easiest sort of medicine to practice. If all you want is a resolution to disease that is rapid and permanent, you really don't need that much skill. Cut it out. Hack it off. Throw it away. Case closed. Even easier, if all you want is a permanent solution, there are many means, successful and unsuccessful, by which this can be achieved. It is often practiced in American medicine, and often leads to a good deal of hand wringing when the doctor has to deliver some difficult news to the patient's survivors. Even when you add rapid to the mix, it isn't all that hard to practice, just don't drag things out too much.

Gentle and permanent, well, that's the basis of many, many forms of complementary and alternative treatments. They go on for years, with massage, change in diet, soothing music and imagery. As long as the disease is not too violent in its actions, or too fast moving, you can do a lot of long-term good moving slowly and gently, if you have a patient who is willing to stay the course of a slow-paced treatment. And, certainly, if circumstances permit, it is likely that, if you change the circumstances of the patient's life to make his environment and lifestyle healthier, a healthier body and patient will ultimately result. But many circumstances, from mechanical injuries to severe pathologies, demand a swifter action on the part of the practitioner. And that's when the practitioner who was just about to light the incense is left with egg on his face.

Rapid and gentle is really, of the three possible pairs of combination, our favorite as a culture. It is all around us. It is the basis of an over-the-counter pharmaceutical industry that makes billions of dollars a year worldwide. As long as the action of the remedy doesn't have to be permanent—which is to say, as long as the medicine does not actually have to do anything other than soothe the patient or his symptoms for a period of time, then it is very easy to have a medical success. But it does not really accomplish anything. The patient is no more well after treatment than he was before. He simply is comforted by something that is gentle in its actions, and, therefore, will not to any great degree actually harm the patient.

But as we have learned in recent years, this is not always the case. Medicines that were promised to safely soothe arthritis pain also were shown to cause heart attacks that killed those same patients. Sleep medications have transformed patients into zombies who eat, talk, and even drive in their sleep without knowing it.

Honestly, it is our addiction to the concept of "rapid and gentle" medicine that is killing us. We have to have better medicine. We deserve better medicine.

We have to not be satisfied with those who would practice medicine that is simply rapid and gentle. Or rapid and permanent. Or gentle and permanent. We have to demand a treatment that is all three: rapid and gentle and permanent.

The whole idea of medicine is that it be rapid. We seek treatment because we are in some sort of discomfort. We need intervention on some physical, mental, or emotional level. And we need it now. A medicine that does not act sufficiently quickly is a medicine that is not effective.

And we have the right that that medicine—the one that is acting quickly—also be gentle. That it should, while it is changing our symptoms and shaping them for our betterment, do no harm. It should in no way be dangerous. And the fact that it is not dangerous should be a proven thing.

Certainly, our government—the agency that we have entrusted to see to it that our medicine is gentle—has failed us time and time again in this matter. And while I in no way defend that government or feel that it has done its job effectively, I feel I must point out that part of this problem is the simple fact that we have, to a great degree, thrown our lot in with allopathic medicine. The suppressive nature of this medicine is, in and of itself, damaging and dangerous. And the fact that allopathic treatments make use of dangerous substances in dangerous doses only increases the problem. If you want medicines that are gentle in their action, then you have to have a benign system of medicine to begin with. And allopathic drugs are, by and large, to no degree benign.

And then there is permanent. When was the last time that a doctor thought that it might be possible for some treatment to actually be permanent in its action? In other words, for it actually to work—to cure something? By this I mean, when was the last time that you really thought that if you got an allopathic treatment that at the end of the treatment your disease would be over, once and for all? Unless that treatment involved a surgery in which the offending part was removed and therefore rendered inert. Or the decay dug out and the tooth filled. Or the bone set and placed in a plaster cast until it healed itself.

Think of how many of our treatments—especially for chronic conditions—involve our going on a medicine and staying on it for the rest of our lives. Dealing with the expense, to say nothing of the potent side effects, for the rest of our lives.

This is certainly true of something as simple as high blood pressure. You will, if you are diagnosed with hypertension, be given some samples of medicines in various combinations until your blood pressure is considered safe. Then your free samples will end and you will have to spend money every month for the rest of your life to continue a treatment that does not in any way cure your condition, only suppresses or controls it. This is also true of allergies, of arthritis, of any number of other chronic conditions.

We have sold our souls to a system of medicine that doesn't even cure us. That only *controls* us by controlling our symptoms.

But again Hahnemann stamps his foot and insists that we have a right as consumers, as patients, as sufferers, to expect a cure that is rapid, gentle, and permanent. And then he went right ahead and established a method of working and a philosophy of thought—both based upon principles that were literally thousands of years old when he codified them—that allowed for all three of those goals to take place and take place simultaneously.

Healing and Curing

One more thing and then we're done. One more definition demanded by Hahnemann's text. It has to do with the first few words of the aphorism. When he speaks of "the highest ideal of cure."

There is a reason why he uses the word "cure," why he does not, within his own medical philosophy, grant the physician the ability to "heal," only the ability—and a lesser thing it is in my own thinking—to "cure." And if I'm wrong about this, if curing is not, as a process and result, a lesser thing than is healing, it is at least something very different.

The difference between healing and curing is the difference between internal and external, and subjective and objective.

The healing process is both internal and subjective. There is something within us, some grace that grants us an innate ability to heal. Something that includes the immune system—that aspect that science has named and, therefore, feels as if to some extent it has mapped out and can manipulate—but extends far beyond it. Hahnemann called this inborn grace "*vital force*." Other forms of alternative medicine call it "*chi*" or "*life force*." The Greeks called it "*dynamus*" from which we have taken the modern word dynamite. It was, therefore, for them an explosive thing.

And, in the same vein, the best allusion that I have seen concerning the healing process is one put forth by Paracelsus, who was in his time about two hundred years before Hahnemann, considered variously to be a madman, a genius, a drug addict, and a healer. Paracelsus said that, for him, the healing process could most effectively and simply be compared to lighting a fire in a fireplace. When you need the heat and light of a fire, you don't have to worry over just how much fire you have to apply to the wood, you simply supply the spark, with the knowledge that the process of combustion is a natural one. That the fire will consume the wood.

In the same way, for Paracelsus, the healing process is a natural one. All that is required is the spark that will allow the healing to begin. That you only have to tend the process like you tend the fire, giving it a gentle poke from time to time. That with healing, as with fire, you have to trust that the process will get it right and will "know what to do." That fire knows all that there is to know about burning—more than you can show it or teach it. In the same way, the healing process within each of us, and open to each of us, is more profound and more capable of transforming our bodies and our beings than anything we can possibly offer by way of enhancement or improvement.

Perhaps what made Paracelsus the healer he proved himself over a lifetime to be was the fact that he knew when *not* to interfere with the healing process. He knew when enough was enough.

Even today, it seems that the mistake that is made again and again in medical treatment—both allopathic and homeopathic—comes from doing too much. We tend to ruin our cases, and spoil our cures when we warp and impede the healing process. And, of course, this is particularly true in allopathic medicine, which simply will not work with the innate healing process, but, instead, desires to change the rules by which we heal. But I have known too many homeopaths who gave too many remedies in too many doses and too many potencies to think that homeopathic medicine is incapable of spoiling the cure, or that it always works within the natural order of healing.

The bottom-line here is that only the patient, only the person who is suffering, can know when and if he is healed. That's what makes it a subjective, as well as an internal, process. Just as we each have a concept of how our body works, how we think, and how we feel when we are well, each of us has a different measuring stick for how we are when we are sick. Therefore, only the patient can truly experience the healing process as it unfolds. And, therefore, the medical practitioner—allopathic or homeopathic—has to listen to and trust the information given him from the patient as to how effective the treatment is and whether or not it is effective.

While the doctor may certainly have objective evidence ranging from blood tests to the witness of his own eyes as to whether or not the patient has been cured, the patient and the patient alone knows whether or not he has been healed. Only he can know if he feels that he has been returned to the state of freedom and health that he enjoyed before the onset of his ills, and only he can give witness to the process as it unfolds. Some will say that they still have the pain, but that they can handle it better. This, surely, is a sign of healing. Others will attest to the ability to do more than they could. And still others will be sleeping better, eating more. Most will, at some point, say that they feel "like themselves." And at this point, the practitioner can know that the healing process is well begun.

The practitioner, in all reality, cannot start the healing process within the patient or stop it or control it. This is beyond the range of medical care. They can, of course, encourage the process, create an environment in which it is more likely to take place, or take place more effectively. That's the whole point of the medicine well selected and well used: Lighting the spark to the fire. But if the wood is wet or if it is unseasoned and not ready to burn, no fire will result. The natural process of combustion cannot take place if it is not begun.

In the same way, if the life force is not sufficient to take the spark, the catalyst of the medicine, then no transformation is possible. This will happen in all our lives. There will be a moment in which there is simply nothing left to burn. In that moment, the life force is snuffed and the life ends. Sadly, the final stage of medical care is always failure. If medical care is created for the sole purpose of restoration of health to those who are ill, then, no matter how many times in a lifespan it works brilliantly, it is destined one day to fail utterly.

But along the way and until this final failure, it is the role of the physician to help tend that flame. This means that physicians should not only be concerned with the restoration of health in times of illness, but also with the maintenance of health in times of strength and health and freedom. The physician must work with the patient before the onset of crisis, to better understand and encourage that patient's ability to heal during times of crisis.

Part of this, most certainly, is in working within natural laws of healing and not against them.

And another part surely has to do with learning to use medicines wisely, both homeopathic and allopathic medicines. We have to find a way to move our culture away from the notion that the daily use of one or more medicines as methods of maintaining order is an acceptable procedure. Medicines work best as catalysts, as sparks that light fires of healing, and not as ongoing modes of suppression that leave the body all the more vulnerable to deeper diseases.

> Medicines work best as catalysts, as sparks that light fires of healing, and not as ongoing modes of suppression that leave the body all the more vulnerable to deeper diseases. . . . And this is, to a great part, what separates "healing" as a process from "curing" as a process.

This is part of our culture's viewpoint—and our doctors'—of what is an acceptable working definition for the word "cure." And this is, to a great part, what separates "healing" as a process from "curing" as a process.

As healing is an internal and subjective process, the ideal of "curing" is both external and objective in nature.

It is external in that the cure is always a *quid pro quo*. A cure is never a simple thing, a clean thing. It often involves an exchange of one symptom for another, or a weakening of the body as a whole in exchange for simple relief from pain. There is always an exchange in terms of symptoms that is implicit in any cure.

Let's illustrate this.

A patient has a clump of symptoms to which we give a group name. That disease diagnosis suggests a group of medicines, and one is selected and given to the patient. The patient's symptoms shift, based on the primary action of that medicine. The doctor looks at the patient once more, and, based upon both his personal experience and his technological testing, he determines that the original symptoms are gone. The patient is, as a result, dismissed from treatment. That is the process of an allopathic cure.

Or a patient has a clump of symptoms. Those symptoms are gathered and examined and a medicine is found from the entire pharmacy of medications available and is selected based upon how closely the total action of the medicines in all the symptoms it is known to create in a state of artificial disease mirrors the natural disease state present in the patient. This is known as the "drug diagnosis." At this point, a required potency for the drug is determined based upon the apparent strength of the patient's vital force and the medicine is given, most often in a single dose. As the medicine begins to work in its primary action, the patient's vital force rises up in reaction to the medicine, and this reactive response triggers the healing process. The practitioner watches and attempts to guide the process, and when that practitioner can determine through objective means (sometimes using the same technological support as does the allopath, sometimes trusting the witness of his own senses) that

the symptoms are gone, the patient is declared cured. This is the process of homeopathic cure.

Either way, it is an external process. The doctor and his medicine are both external forces acting upon the internal being of the patient. Either way, it is intrusive, to a
greater or lesser degree. This is the process of cure.

It is also objective. While only the patient may know if he really and truly feels
that he has been healed and made whole, the doctor is much better suited to gathering objective or scientific proof as to the success or failure of treatment.

Both processes—healing and curing—are therefore valuable and each has its
place. When we fuse the healing process with a wise external influence, we get a
dynamic result. But when the potency of the two processes becomes lopsided—most
especially when the aspect of cure dominates the process of healing—then disaster is
likely to result. Part of the problem with modern allopathic (and, unfortunately, some
homeopathic) medicine is that the healing process has been left behind in the mix.
This is especially unfortunate in that so much of allopathic medicine, as I have said
before, simply attempts to buy time while depending upon the body's own innate ability to heal to get the job done. So, at once the allopath depends upon and works
against the body's ability to heal itself. No wonder we are all so very sick.

Let's get back to Hahnemann. When he talks about the "highest ideal of cure,"
he is recognizing that the role of the physician is an external and objective role. The
doctor cannot become the patient, cannot experience firsthand what the patient is
experiencing. Nor should he. If the doctor is not objective, then he is useless. The
role of the doctor, and of the physician, is to cure—to act as that outside catalyst that
can help the patient's own innate healing process to spring to life and to return that
patient to health.

To continue with the aphorism, it is also the role of the physician to be a catalyst
whose action it is to be rapid, gentle, and permanent in working against the disease
and for the life of the patient. Both things at once. To be effective, the physician must
find a way to rid the patient of a disease and to help restore his health, a way that is
gentle and does no harm. A way that works quickly enough that health be restored
before that disease can do real damage or kill the patient. And a way that actually
works—that once the treatment is completed and health is restored, health can also
be maintained.

I said at the beginning of this chapter that, with this simple aphorism, Hahnemann set the bar high, both for the responsibility of the physician and the expectation of the patient. I also said that, after making such a dynamic statement, he then
actually set about creating the method of working that would allow a physician to
achieve these goals.

The rest of this book will explore that method of working.

Learning and Unlearning: Getting from Allopathy to Homeopathy

"You will see the old grandfather sit off in a corner of the room, and if he sees little Johnnie running towards him, he will say, 'Oh, do keep away, keep away.' Give him a dose of Arnica and he will let Johnnie run all over him."

—J. T. KENT IN LECTURES ON HOMEOPATHIC MATERIA MEDICA

CHAPTER FIVE

What Arnica
Has to Tell Us

A few years back, when I was still leading my first study group here in Connecti-cut, I was invited to take part in a gathering of New England study groups. I happily traveled to a small town in Massachusetts to a motel of some sort for what turned out to be rather a homeopathic Jamboree.

This was a daylong event, during which a number of homeopathic practition-ers—naturopathic physicians all, if I remember correctly—came to speak to us about homeopathy. We then gathered as group leaders to discuss how to teach homeopathy.

One of the speakers was a homeopathic practitioner from Connecticut, who, like me had crossed the state line for the meeting. I am sure that as he stood in front of us, happy-faced and clueless crew that we were, he was struck with the notion that he had better give this group a strong dose of homeopathic philosophy before loosing us once more upon the unsuspecting public.

So I remember that, as he stood there in front of us, behind that cheesy motel podium in his ancient tweed jacket, he took a minute and thought about what he was about to say before he said it.

Finally he bore into the group with an electric blue gaze and then said, "Do you all know that Arnica is not a remedy for bruises?" or something to that effect.

The response to this surprised me, even then. I would have expected shock or laughter, either being appropriate responses from those who were being told some-thing that challenged their beliefs, or was so elementary as to make them wonder why they had traveled to come to this meeting.

No, the crowd reacted as if the speaker had said something rude, or as if he had stood behind the particleboard podium and loudly passed gas. And, like gas, the speaker's comments just hung there, poisoning the air for a long moment. A moment in which everyone seemed to be looking at their shoes.

Then all hell broke loose. Hands went up in the air from those who, while pas-sionate, were still willing to play by Scout rules. Others, more passionate or less polite, just started speaking at once. Some were asking questions. Others were making comments about what they had heard.

All from that little sentence. That little sentence that said all at once, "You have been thinking this, but you are wrong to think it." And, "You have been teaching this, and you are wrong to teach it."

You see, to a bunch of study group leaders, most of whom, like me at that time, were just staying a page ahead of their students in whatever book they were using as their text, this little sentence pretty much would have pulled the rug out from under us if the rug underfoot hadn't been one of those green, geometric-patterned, wall-to-wall motel rugs that hide stains and cause vertigo to all those who stand staring at their feet.

Yes, to those of us at the jamboree, this was heady stuff. Perhaps, we were being told, we should have read something beyond a paperback home guide to homeopathic remedies before we started the study group. Perhaps we shouldn't be teaching it at all.

In retrospect, I think that all the speaker was really trying to do was get a gauge of exactly our level of understanding and expertise. I think that I would give him too much credit for insight and wisdom if I were to suspect that he had any indication of what the response would be before he began speaking. And given that, after the initial explosion died down, he found himself looking, for the rest of his speech, at crossed arms and stone faces, I tend to think that I am right in my assessment.

But, however inadvertent, the speaker had said something important. Something that I say to you right now: you do know by now that Arnica is not the homeopathic remedy for bruises, don't you?

If not, go back and read Part One another time, because you missed something important.

Think of the Grand Canyon. Think of how distinct the distance is between the sides of the canyon and how deep the divide. It is surely death to anyone who would, like Thelma and Louise, attempt to leap, or drive, across the canyon.

Now think of the words "homeopathy" and "allopathy." Picture them in capital letters, floating in space. Now insert the Grand Canyon between those two words. And you have a realistic assessment of how homeopathy is related to allopathy.

Those who want to cling to the idea that Arnica is a remedy for bruises are still clinging to allopathic thinking. And, if you are to study homeopathy, practice homeopathy or, God forbid, dedicate your life to teaching it, then you are going to have to change your thinking.

See, the mistake that too many people make—students and practitioners alike—is that they change their pharmaceuticals, but not their thinking. And they have to change their thinking.

If you are to learn homeopathy, then you have to unlearn allopathy somewhere along the way. You are going to have to let go of this ritualistic form of medicine that has been beaten into your head since you listened in on the conversations your mother had with her doctor while you were still in the womb. You are going to have to give up the colorful liquids and pills and all hope that there is some actual merit in the phrase "new and improved."

You are going to have to change your thinking.

To still be thinking that Arnica is a bruise remedy is to still be believing that diseases are invaders in our bodies, that there is some way for a medicine to get between that disease and our bodies in order to put things right. You are going to have to come to see that the symptoms that we associate with disease are our bodies' responses to catalysts and stresses of all sorts, and that the diseases that plague us *are* us, and that we *are* our diseases. That's why, with the exception of epidemics, we each of us tends to experience a specific illness in a very specific and unique way. That's why, no matter how infectious the disease, there will always be someone who just plain does not cooperate with the allopathic model and get sick when they come into contact with the infectious agent. That's why some of us are still sick by other people's standards when we consider ourselves to be healthy, while others are positively robust from our point of view when they consider themselves to be sick.

> You are going to have to come to see that the symptoms that we associate with disease are our bodies' responses to catalysts and stresses of all sorts, and that the diseases that plague us *are* us, and that we *are* our diseases.

In order to work with disease in a new way—one that will hopefully prove itself in your own life to be more valuable in creating and maintaining a state of true good health—you have to first come to think about disease in a new way. And then you have to come to think about health and attaining and maintaining health in a new way.

This is the process that I call *unlearning*. It does not involve just one light bulb going on over your head. No, it will involve so many bulbs flashing that you will think that you are on a red carpet.

To be still thinking that Arnica is a bruise remedy is to totally miss the point of homeopathy: that you can't treat a bruise, or a cold or cancer, you can only treat the person with a bruise, a cold or cancer. You can only work with their symptoms and, by giving an appropriate remedy, whose power it is to mimic the natural symptoms already in place, allow for that healing spark that can send the weakened, stuck, and ill patient on a journey toward healing.

And to still be thinking that Arnica is a bruise remedy is to underestimate the possibilities that Arnica represents. If you are foolish enough to cling to the idea that Arnica is only good for children who have fallen off their swings and gotten a booboo, then you are missing so much potential for healing in your own life and in the lives of those you love.

What Arnica Does

Arnica was one of the very first homeopathic remedies ever created. And given that most of the early homeopathic remedies were taken from herbal medicines whose potential for healing had already been proven tried and true, it should come as no surprise to anyone that Arnica would be in the first handful of herbal medicines that became homeopathic remedies.

As an herbal medicine, Arnica was so well known in the ancient world that the physicians attending the injured in the Roman army made use of the Arnica plant.

The Arnica plant is native to mountain regions, especially to the Alps. Its German name is "Fallkraut" and, just as it sounds, it received this name due to its known affinity to the injuries associated with the effects of falls.

As both an herbal medicine, and as a homeopathic, it has been associated with the treatment of pain, most especially with the pain resulting from mechanical injury.

But for those who take their knowledge of homeopathic remedies from the Materia Medica, and not from paperback home guides to homeopathy, there is a good deal more to understand about the use of even as simple and elementary remedy as Arnica.

You see, in addition to the symptoms that each remedy would be said to have the ability to treat, each remedy has a set of modalities. Modalities, as will be discussed in more detail in the chapters ahead, are the catalysts that make each of these symptoms feel better or worse. Through a thorough understanding of the modalities of each symptom, the practitioner is able to select the remedy that has been shown not only to be effective in treating patients with a given symptom, but also with similar modalities of that symptom. Therefore, it is not enough to say that Arnica is effective in cases in which the patient has suffered some form of mechanical injury, most especially if that injury has resulted in bruising of the body, we have to also say that this is a patient who has undergone a mechanical injury and, as a result is bruised and refuses to let anyone touch his body. This modality of being worse from being touched is key to identifying the need for Arnica.

The patient who needs Arnica will often be in a state of shock. In fact, Arnica is one of our best remedies for those who are in shock. And this shock need not have come about as a result of mechanical injury. The shock could result from bad news, from emotional upset as well. Arnica has often been used to help those who were coping with the loss of a loved one, or other severe emotional trauma. It has been an important remedy in helping victims of rape or victims of violent robbery. It has been used for patients suffering long-term effects of violence and can be effective years after the event, whether the trauma was physical or emotional in nature or both. It has even been used for those who have had a terrible nightmare and who need soothing before they can return to sleep. In fact, Arnica can be used successfully in cases of chronic insomnia, as long as the pattern of the illness matches the pattern of the remedy.

Arnica should even be considered in cases in which the patient is suffering from overwork. When the patient's system has finally become overwhelmed by stress or responsibility.

Here is a person that, due to some shocking emotional or physical event, will often be completely out of touch with their situation. Thus, he will attempt to send the doctor away, although the doctor is very much needed. He will insist that there is nothing wrong with him. He will, of course, refuse to be examined and will not be touched.

For people needing Arnica, touch is a major issue. Their whole body becomes overly sensitive. Their sense of touch has been altered through their trauma, so that everything overwhelms them as concerns the sense of touch. Thus, you will often have a "Princess and the Pea" syndrome, in which even their bed's mattress will suddenly be too hard. And the patients needing Arnica—from here, let's just call them "Arnica patients" for simplicity's sake—will toss and turn, unable to find a comfortable position.

Not only are they worse from touch, they are also worse for motion, most specifically for any jarring motion, any sudden motion. This remedy may be very useful for those who have suddenly overexerted. For those who decide to take an exercise class after years of sedentary living. For those who hurry to work in their gardens after winter months in which they did not bend and kneel. It is an excellent remedy for women suffering the pains associated with childbirth, and for the recovery period after childbirth.

It is, in fact, an excellent remedy to consider whenever any form of surgery is required. Many practitioners will insist (allopathically, I may point out) that anyone undergoing surgery should take the remedy both before and after the surgery as a matter of routine. And, most certainly, a dose or two of Arnica before surgery can surely do no harm. And after surgery, it is a matter of seeing how the body reacts to the trauma of surgery before selecting among the most common post-surgical remedies, including Arnica, as well as Staphysagria, Hypericum, and Phosphorus, among many others.

Emotionally, the Arnica patient will feel wounded as well. Although they say they need no help, and certainly will not let themselves be touched, they will often say that they feel like a wounded animal.

Also, the Arnica type will seem disoriented. They may even seem unconscious or partially conscious. But, if you call them by name or ask them a question, they will often rouse themselves to answer you. It may be as if they are on a seven-second delay, and you will sometimes see them pull back into consciousness in direct response to your voice, but they will answer you. They often will drift off once more.

This can be a nervous patient, and a very fearful one. They may fear that they are about to die. But, fearful as they are, they know that they want to be left alone. Look for the Arnica patient—especially those with a chronic need for Arnica based upon a deep emotional trauma—to be fearful of open spaces. They may fear the mall, fear crowds; they may even refuse to leave their house.

This is a very important remedy for those who have suffered strokes and for those with severe head injuries. It can be a very important remedy for the elderly.

Think of Arnica in cases of influenza that follow the general pattern here. Think of Arnica in cases of bleeding, hemorrhaging in any part of the body. This is certainly true in cases of hemorrhage that are brought on by mechanical injury. But you would sell the remedy short if you thought of it only for hemorrhages that were brought on by mechanical injury.

This is an important remedy for heart and circulatory conditions as well. It is useful in cases of angina or palpitations in which the patient will feel his whole body shaken by his pounding heart, and for patients with pain in the region of the heart that travels from left to right. It can be especially useful for those who suffer nightmares or night terror that is accompanied by heart pain or palpitations.

Therefore, it can be said that Arnica can be useful for something as simple as a black eye and something as complex and threatening as heart disease. Among its other clinical uses are: abscesses and boils of all sort, chronic pain, headache and back pain, most especially when it is associated with stress or injury. It can be a remedy for those with diabetes, for those with flu, with whooping cough or with dysentery. As a remedy associated with blood and, especially, with reabsorption of blood (you should first think of bruises and bruising, which is a gathering of blood under the skin—the healing process here is a reabsorption process), it is a remedy for those with the skin condition known as purpura. It is an excellent remedy for those with sprains, especially those with old sprains that tend to reinjure over time again and again. It is a great remedy for those with rheumatic pains and lumbago, when the pattern of the pain follows the pattern of the remedy's action. It can even be a remedy for those two great traumas of middle-aged men: baldness and impotence.

Now, let's deal with an important issue here. A question that I have been asked again and again over the years. I have listed many different uses for this one medicine. And I have only given a partial list, believe me. There is much more to know about his remedy. Whole books have been written about Arnica.

So, Arnica does a whole lot of things, works in a lot of ways. But do you need to have all these symptoms in order for this to be the right remedy for you?

The answer is simple: no. You don't need to have baldness and impotence in order for this to be an appropriate remedy. Instead, turn that thinking around—if you have baldness, impotence, or both, then you should consider this among the remedies that might be right for you. And to determine which remedy is the right one, you have to do what you always have to do, you have to match the symptoms and modalities that you are experiencing with the symptoms and modalities that the remedy manifests in "well" people.

Like every other homeopathic remedy, Arnica has been tested again and again. Healthy people have been given the remedy and have, in a double-blind study, kept specific records on the changes that the medicine created. And the remedy is not tested just on one person, but on many, so that the power of the remedy in a wide population can be recognized and known. So that when the remedy is given there are no surprises, no side effects, and toxic outcome.

So, to think of Arnica as the remedy for bruises, is not only inappropriate—which is to say allopathic—it is also to sell this remedy short. And, as a result, such thinking will guide you to leave the remedy on the shelf when you should be rushing for it.

Oh, one last note—I couldn't fit this in anywhere else, but it needs saying. Arnica is available at health-food stores as both a topical and an internal remedy. It comes in pill form, like all the other remedies, but is also available in rubs and creams. And these topical forms can be very useful in cases of sprains or overexertion. But please remember that Arnica must never be used topically on any open wound, any cut or scrape. Now, if you make a mistake and use Arnica topically on a scrape, you won't kill anyone, but it will hurt like hell, and you will only make that mistake once. Other remedies, like Calendula, are wonderful to soothe and inspire healing from open wounds. Just don't apply Arnica topically whenever the skin is broken or cut.

Oh, and one other thing—about those bruises. You can't even walk away from this text thinking that Arnica is the only bruise remedy. It will not—I repeat, it will not—work for bruises if the case does not match the remedy. And it is far from the only homeopathic remedy that will heal those who have been bruised by mechanical injury. If you look in your repertory under the rubric of "bruises," you're going to find forty-four different remedies. So, to jump to the conclusion that because the patient has a bruise he or she needs Arnica is just plain sloppy and dumb. They may need Sulphur, or Phosphorus, or Ledum—such a great remedy for sprained ankles or black eyes, even bug bites that follow the Ledum pattern—or Bryonia or Calcarea Carbonica, which is great for bruises that don't want to heal, or Bellis Perennis, which is excellent for deep bruising that Arnica can't always cure and, therefore, is an excellent follow-up remedy for Arnica in mechanical injury. The list of potential remedies just goes on and on.

And each of these remedies, like Arnica, has its own story to tell, it own modalities and symptoms, its own way of being, each of which represents an attempt at healing. If you can remember that the symptoms are not caused by the disease itself, but are, rather, your body's attempt to react to and heal from that disease, then you can begin to see each remedy's pattern of symptoms as that specific strategy of healing. And in doing so, you can begin to better understand where each remedy is "coming from" (to get a little anthropomorphic), and its specific path of healing. If you can get to this point, then you will be able to differentiate Calcarea's path in healing a bruise from Arnica's. And the selection of the appropriate remedy in the appropriate circumstance for the appropriate patient will get all the easier.

What Arnica Has to Tell Us

So what are you to take away from this mishmash of study group jamborees and severe blows to the head? What does Arnica have to tell us?

It first reminds us of something that we will tend to forget if we don't change our way of thinking—that no medicine, whether it is a simple acute remedy with limited medicinal value or a deeply transformational polycrest remedy, does only one thing. That's a mistake that allopaths make; they do not apply their knowledge of all the actions that a medicine takes with equal understanding, but, instead, attempt to separate primary actions from side effects, which is both ridiculous and foolhardy. Foolhardy because they could make better use of their own medicines if they used them to their full potential by manipulating their full value.

And it tells us that we can never underestimate the full value of any remedy by limiting in our minds what it can do, or under which circumstances it might be of value.

In the same way, Arnica reminds us that we must never in homeopathic medicine, limit our remedies in other ways, which is to say that we cannot allow ourselves to ever think allopathically, even in moments of crisis. We can never associate a given remedy with a given single symptom, no matter how often or how effectively it works for that single symptom. Even if it is the remedy of choice 99 percent of the time, you may be faced with

> The core of what Arnica is trying to tell us is this: homeopathy is fundamentally different from allopathic medicine. Therefore, it is fundamentally different from what we grew up thinking medicine is.

that 1 percent, that one patient in one hundred for whom it will not work.

To call Arnica a "bruise remedy" is to both underestimate the full value of the remedy and to underestimate the many (forty-four, to be exact) ways in which a bruise may be dealt with by the body as it attempts to heal that bruise.

The core of what Arnica is trying to tell us is this: homeopathy is fundamentally different from allopathic medicine. Therefore, it is fundamentally different from what we grew up thinking medicine is. It's like we suddenly find ourselves on a soap opera and are being told that the man we grew up thinking was our father is not our father after all. And worse, our real father is a poor pathetic guy who has no money and no respect in Pine Valley. And yet this is the man to whom we owe our life.

No, Arnica—by the way it works and by the fact that it works so very efficiently—is telling us that homeopathy is not allopathy. That homeopathic medicines are not allopathic and should not be used allopathically. That those who would be homeopaths cannot allow themselves to think allopathically, even in the most dire situations.

And finally Arnica concludes that, no, it is not the remedy for bruises.

PART TWO

Homeopathy

"There are just two main modes of medical treatment, the homeopathic and the allopathic. The homeopathic mode bases all that it
does on the exact observation of nature, careful experiments, and
pure experience. It was never, before me, been intentionally applied.
The allopathic (or heteropathic) mode does not do this. Each mode
is diametrically opposed to the other. Only a person who does not
know both could surrender to the delusion that they could ever
approach one another, let alone ever let themselves be united. Only
such a person could make himself so ridiculous as to practice sometimes homeopathically and sometimes allopathically, according to
the pleasure of the patient. Such a practice may be called a treason-
ous betrayal of divine homeopathy."

—SAMUEL HAHNEMANN IN THE *ORGANON OF MEDICINE*

CHAPTER SIX

The Magic Spark

If we at long last are going to talk about homeopathy, then we are going to have to stop talking about substance and start talking about energy. Stop thinking about leaves and start thinking about sparks.

And to understand the concept of homeopathy as energy medicine—far closer to acupuncture in its action than to herbal medicine—we have to first understand that Samuel Hahnemann was a vitalist.

The Vitalist Viewpoint

By "vitalist" I mean that Hahnemann believed the fact that the earth and all that is natural to it is alive. And not in a benign "spring is coming again, here come the first flowers pushing their heads through the melting snow" kind of way. No, nature—or, more correctly, Nature, because the vitalist cannot help but find some sort of persona or intellect present—is a wilder, more untamable thing. For the vitalist, the ecosystem within which we exist is a throbbing thing. Ever changing and ever growing. For the vitalist, Nature responds to human perception and human will by evolving, by mutating. Therefore, we live within a realm of catalyst and response, creation and destruction, of will butting up against will. It is a wild thing, an unknowable thing—or, at best, only partly knowable—the nature of Nature.

For the vitalist, creation imbued a life-spark within all that was created. Therefore, the animals, the plants, the rocks and water, all share an aspect of creation and an aspect of life, each evolving, each mutating and changing into ever more successful creatures. Creatures that are ever more distinct in their sense of self.

So, for the vitalist, the aspect within any medicine, homeopathic or allopathic, that makes it medicinal is the life spark itself. In taking a medicine, we are digesting the life energy of another aspect of creation, one whose own evolution gave it a survival strategy that we now need to "borrow" in order to be well. This would be why the vitalist would argue that natural medicines, either herbal or homeopathic in nature, are far more desirable than technological medicines, since most modern medicines are chemically produced, or, at best, highly refined, and are therefore lacking in this life energy upon which we are all dependant for our very survival. Just as with food, they would argue, when we refine our medicines, we take them a step away from being of true value within our systems. The vitalist would argue that we are, whether we like it or not, animals, and, as such, respond best to things that speak directly to our animal nature, which is to say that the closer it comes from being ripped from the ground by our own hand, the better.

> . . . the aspect within any medicine, homeopathic or allopathic, that makes it medicinal is the life spark itself. In taking a medicine, we are digesting the life energy of another aspect of creation, one whose own evolution gave it a survival strategy that we now need to "borrow" in order to be well.

So, for medical practitioners who, like Hahnemann, are vitalists, it is important that this medicinal life spark be used in a manner that is at the same time most beneficial and most powerful. This is a hard blend, especially if you are trying to stay as true as possible to the natural state.

This need for the practitioner to find a medicine that was at one time safe and effective was perhaps the major force that drove Hahnemann in the development of homeopathy. As he studied and practiced medicine more than two hundred years ago, he worked with a group of commonly used medicines that included such things as arsenic. Medicines that, perhaps because they were imbued with such a powerful life spark, most certainly had impact upon the patient's life, but in no way could be called benign or safe for use.

Even after Hahnemann had himself evolved to the point of understanding that medicines worked more effectively if they worked with symptoms and not against them, he still was faced with the very real problem of the toxicity of the medicines themselves.

With his philosophy of what would someday be called homeopathy in place, Samuel Hahnemann set about developing a way in which that philosophy could embody in a practice of medicine that would be both safe and effective.

The Healing Enigma

Faced with the same situation, what would you do? You have been trained as a doctor, taught the use of the medicines on hand. And yet, you have seen over and over again that these things that are called medicine, that are supposed to help patients who are weak or sick or in pain, create more problems than they solve. Even before he finished medical school, it had become apparent to Samuel Hahnemann that the medicines that he had been taught to use in the restoration of health were, in reality toxic. He saw that more patients were dying from their cures than were dying from their diseases.

So, you are faced with the same dilemma—the medicine that you have been trained to use is toxic, it quite literally poisons the patients. But there is no other form of medicine available. What you have been taught to do is all that is known about medicine. And yet, it is not good enough, it does not do the job. So, what do you do?

First, you go with logic. If a medicinal substance is too toxic for use in its natural form, you dilute it. Mix it with water. Or, if it won't dissolve in water, you try grinding it and grinding it and grinding it and then mixing it with an inert powdery substance until it will dissolve. The thinking is, if this much is poisonous, perhaps less will still have some medicinal punch, but won't be quite so toxic.

It's a simple enough principle and it requires a lot of trial and error. Just how much is still too much—still toxic? And how much is just too diluted, too weak to act medicinally?

This could drive you crazy. Working and working and working in such a way that, once you have found the correct level for one substance you can reproduce it, not only with that substance, but with other toxins.

And remember, it's not good if you can only do it once. It has to work again and again in case after case.

So remember to keep good notes. And to set up some sort of system so that you can always be sure that the level of dilution is exactly the same from dose to dose of the same medicine and from medicine to medicine.

This is, after all, one of the greatest weaknesses of herbal medicine. In that two leaves of the same plant could be more or less potent than each other, to say nothing of two crops in the same field, much less many different plants grown in many different places, many different soils over a period of years, it can be very hard to be sure that two tinctures, two teas, or two poultices will have exactly the same medicinal punch. And this is part of the toxic problem, after all. Two digitalis plants may, because of their differing potencies, have different effects—one medicinal and the other toxic.

So part of the problem facing Hahnemann was not only that the medicines were toxic, but also that they were, if you will forgive the wording, not *reliably* toxic. You just could not be sure exactly how powerful they were until you used them, and by then it could be too late.

So the issue of toxicity in the use of medicines in their natural form had two parts—the toxic nature of the substances and the unreliability of their potency. In solving one, you have to solve the other as well.

This means that if you are going to dilute the substances, you have to dilute them systematically.

The system of dilution, as Hahnemann created it, took 1 part of a substance and mixed it with 99 parts water or other dissolving medium. This scale is referred to as the "C" scale, "C" being the Roman numeral for "100." This scale is, of course, infinite in nature, in that you can always add another level of dilution. You can always take one level of dilution and take it to the next level by mixing it again with 99 parts of water.*

The homeopathic remedies that you buy today in health-food stores are grouped according to potency, which reflects the level of dilution for that particular remedy. Thus, a 1C potency has only one level of dilution, while a 12C has a dozen levels. And the 30C potency has always gone through thirty levels of dilution.

The other scale of dilution that has been established is the "X" scale, named for the Roman numeral for "10." In this, 1 part of the original substance is mixed with 9 parts dissolving medium.

This scale of dilution, while it produces a medicinal product that is perfectly homeopathic in both nature and action, is not Hahnemann's own creation. Instead, it is attributed variously to three of Hahnemann's contemporaries, chief among them is Constantin Hering.

As a simple rule of thumb, it should be noted that the C scale can be considered twice as dilute as the X scale, since 10 X 10 = 100. So a 30C potency of a given homeopathic medicine would have approximately the same dilution as would a 60X potency of the same medicine.

But dilution is not potency. It is simply a matter of mathematics, how much substance has been dissolved in how much water.

The enigma that is central to homeopathic medicine has to do with the relationship between dilution and potency.

Common sense would tell us that the X scale, that which is closer to the original substance in its full organic strength, should be medicinally more potent than the remedies of the C scale, which are far more diluted, far further away in chemical composition from the original substance.

And this is where homeopathy begins to defy common sense.

Hahnemann found in his experiments that, again and again, as the remedies became more and more diluted, they became both more powerful medicinally, that is, more capable of acting as a catalyst, and less toxic. Over and over he found that, at a certain level of dilution, all toxicity stopped. Today we know that at that level all of

---

* At the level of 1,000 dilutions, however, the scale takes on the Roman numeral for 1,000 and becomes the "M" scale. The scale of dilution is the same, only the letter changes.

the molecules of the original substance have fallen away, so there is nothing left that *can* be toxic.* Hahnemann did not, in his day, have the technology to know exactly why this was happening. He could only note, based upon his empirical experience, that it did.

In that homeopaths both in Hahnemann's day and after, were quite aware that the more diluted a remedy became, the more powerful it seemed to be as a catalyst to healing encouraged two early homeopaths Professor Hugo Schulz and Dr. H. R. Arndt to do enough research to develop what is today known as the Arndt-Schulz Law. The fact that both of these men, who publicly were considered to be allopathic doctors, were in all actuality closeted homeopaths must surely be forgiven.

Simply put, the Arndt-Schulz Law—also called the "Biphasal Paradoxical Effect" by those wishing to truly dazzle you with their words—states that small or gentle catalysts enhance the growth of living things, while medium-strength catalysts allow for status quo and stronger catalysts inhibit or destroy growth. As with Hahnemann's observations, the Arndt-Schulz Law is based upon empirical observation.

Over the years, the Arndt-Schulz Law has been tested and questioned. Among those to do so was a French homeopath known as Meyhoffer, who is quoted by homeopath and author William Boericke in his *Pocket Manual of Homeopathic Materia Medica* as writing, "From the moment a drug produces pathogenetic symptoms, it exaggerates the function of the tissue, exhausts the already diminished vitality, and thence, instead of stimulating the organic cell in the direction of life, impairs or abolishes its power of contraction." In other words, that which pushes against a symptom and suppresses it with the sheer toxic strength of a particular medicine not only fails to cure the condition, but also manages to weaken the system as a whole, leaving it all the more vulnerable, not only to the original disease, but also to a plethora of other conditions.

There is no way to overstate the importance of this discovery. With as simple an

---

* This level of dilution is constant at 12C or 23X. On either scale of dilution this is the point at which no molecules of the original substance remain. This level of dilution is called "Avogadro's Number," in honor of Amadeo Avogadro (1776–1856), an Italian chemist who was both a revolutionary and reviled in his field as Hahnemann was in medicine. Although the two of them were coming to about the same conclusions at roughly the same time, it is not known whether they were aware of each other's work. Over time, Avogadro's Number has proven to be a bit off. In fact, only a few years after he came up with his number, it was slightly improved upon by a physicist named Josef Loschmidt (1821–1895). For this reason, fans of Loschmidt's work insist upon calling this level of dilution the "Loschmidt Number."

In proving that Avogadro in his day got no more respect and support from his contemporaries than Hahnemann did, it should be noted that, after he was hounded and jeered for years because of his findings, Avogadro's Number was accepted as scientific fact only four years after his death.

act as dilution, Hahnemann had managed to discover a method in which medicines could not only be made safe, but one in which they could actually be made more powerful and more effective as well. And, in that you can always take the medicine to another level of dilution, the remedies could be made infinitely more powerful as needed.

At the same time, Hahnemann had also, with his two different scales of dilution, solved the problem of consistency. While one medicine may be found to work more effectively at a higher or lower level of dilution than did another, both doctor and patient could be quite sure that a 12C is a 12C is a 12C, with no exceptions.

Hahnemann had therefore, in his practice of medicine, made two huge discoveries. First, thanks to that chinchona bark, he had realized that medicines work better when they are used to stimulate symptoms and not suppress them. And second, he had discovered that he could make his medicines both safer and more powerful by diluting them. He still didn't have a name for what he was doing, but he knew that he was onto something by doing it over and over again.

Now what happened next may well be apocryphal. But if it is, if it truly didn't happen historically, well, then it should have, because it is just a great story.*

Picture Hahnemann as he practiced medicine. As doctors of his day traveled to their patients and as Hahnemann practiced medicine in a rural region of Germany, he spent a good part of his day going from farm to farm in a little wooden horse-drawn cart. He rode on a hard wooden seat in the front of his cart. And in the back were Hahnemann's medicines. He had to take them with him because, after all, he had made them himself. They were not available anywhere else. So his cart was filled with diluted, and, therefore, liquid medicines, all sloshing around in their corked glass bottles.

Now as with any other doctor, I am sure that Hahnemann would often, as he made his rounds, see many cases of a particular cold or flu that was making the rounds of his region. Therefore, he would often be treating the same condition in several patients on the same day. And he, therefore, would often make use of the same medi-

---

* Please note that this story did not happen. It is a homeopathic myth that has been told again and again over the generations. Homeopathic historian Julian Winston has told me that Hahnemann had neither horse nor carriage and that, if he did see patients in their own homes, he had to walk. Historically, Hahnemann experimented with dilutions between 1811 and 1819. In these years, he began using sugar granules as a means of holding his liquid potencies. He actually began to success the remedies to, as he put it, "get a uniform mixture." I thank Julian for his knowledge and beg the reader not to believe a word of anecdote about the wagon. I include it here only because it is my particular favorite, what with Hahnemann taking his wagon through the Hartz Mountains, and the jingle-jangle of the remedies as the horse made his way along his daily route. It's a sweet story, and I am a great believer in mythology. So appreciate it only as a myth, and not as historical fact.

cine in different patients on the same day. All from the liquids in the corked glass bottles.

Over time as he used his medicines again and again, Hahnemann noticed that the patients who received their dose of medicine at the end of the day seemed to get more benefit from their medication than did those who got theirs at the beginning of the day. It was as if the medicines, simply by traveling in the rickety little cart, were growing stronger and stronger.

As this story goes, it was this simple observation that lead Samuel Hahnemann to the second component in the creation of homeopathic remedies—succussion.

Succussion is nothing more than shaking. The remedy in liquid form is shaken quite vigorously at each level of dilution. And each shake ends with a jolt. Now, over the years, I have been taught that that "jolt" was the slapping of the vial against everything from the shaker's other hand to the cover of a leather-bound Bible. But it doesn't really matter what exactly was used to slam the remedy against. The point is, the remedies are not just diluted, but shaken as well and shaken systematically. Just as each dilution must always be exactly the same—so that each 6C has exactly the same level of dilution—in the same way, each remedy must also be succussed in the same way.

Stop Making Sense

The question remains as to just why the remedies get less toxic while they are more and more diluted, while, at the same time, become more and more powerful as medicinal agents.

There is no set answer to this question. I tend to think that, just as Hahnemann in his day lacked the technology to show that a 30C dose of Arsenicum has not a single trace of toxic arsenic, we today lack the technology that would prove to all that the so-called microdoses of homeopathic remedies contain a potent form of energy.

But until we have a machine that will measure life energy or vital force, I have a theory that may well hold us over.

I believe, as I have said before, that all medicines in their actions make use of the vital force that was originally present in the source material, animal, vegetable or mineral, and transfer a portion of that energy to the patient who ingests the medicine. This vital force is never toxic, no matter the source material of the medicine, because it is the animating and regenerating force within all living things. What can be quite toxic is the actual substance, whether it be vegetable material like the poison ivy plant, or mineral substance like arsenic, or animal material, such as snake venom. All three of these materials become powerful homeopathic remedies once they have been diluted and succussed, through the process known as *potentization*.

What the potentizing process does in removing the actual material nature of the original substance is remove anything that can be toxic to other creatures. At the same time, as the substance falls away in the process of creating a homeopathic remedy, the vital force that was innate within that substance remains.

As I have said in earlier pages, I believe that when we take a medicine of any sort—allopathic or homeopathic, substance-based or energy-based—we are borrowing the vital force contained within that medicine, and, along with it, the evolutionary plan of that species. Its survival skills, if you will. This might well explain why one particular herb might be very useful for a specific disease of the human eye. Why would one herb—horse chestnut, for example—be of use to the human eye and not another? Some might say because the one herb contains a particular chemical compound unique to it. But why does this herb contain this particular chemical compound? Something allowed it to evolve that way, something that can only be part of Nature. If you believe, as I do, and as most vitalists must surely believe, that Nature is guided by some sort of intelligence, then it makes sense that that intelligence was also at work in the evolutionary process itself. That there is some reason why that particular plant contains that particular, useful compound.

From the moment that man began intervening as his fellow man fell victim to disease, he had to turn to the world around him, to the plants, animals, and minerals that were part of his local environment, in order to find something that he would one day call medicine. If the plants and animals and, yes, even the minerals around us were not part and parcel of the same creation that created the human race, then these things could not be used to assist us in our time of need. It is because we are all part of the same system, the same creation, that we share the common bond of vital force that these medicines work for us at all.

And it is this common life spark, this vital force that is itself the catalyst to healing.

When the substance is potentized into a homeopathic remedy it loses the toxic "shell" of substance. At the same time, the vital force becomes more focused, more direct in its action. It is as if you were dialing in a radio station on an old analog radio. As you moved the dial closer and closer to the station, the signal would become clearer and clearer. The sounds of static and of other stations would ultimately disappear as you tuned into your station. Finally, you were left with just the one station and a clear signal. In the same way, as you potentize the remedy, you clear away the static of the substance and allow the clear signal to play through. The more and more diluted it becomes, the clearer and clearer the signal and the more direct and powerful the action of the remedy.

In taking a homeopathic remedy you are borrowing the vital force of another living thing, whether it is a plant, an animal, or a mineral. In the pages ahead, we will look at how these three categories of substance each yield a group of remedies with common traits and common actions within the human system.

But, for now, the point is this: that the vital force of the remedy contains, as I see it, the survival strategy of the original substance. By this I do not mean the survival strategy of the individual plant, animal, or mineral from which the sample of substance was taken, but of the group strategy that allowed this aspect of creation to change, grow and survive throughout the evolutionary process.

This is important, because this strategy contains a map of sorts, an energy that speaks to our own vital force. And this map shows a pathway to healing. If that path is congruent with our own, if the vital force of the remedy speaks to our own, then healing takes place. If it does not, if they cannot communicate together, then healing does not take place.

> This strategy contains a map of sorts, an energy that speaks to our own vital force. And this map shows a pathway to healing. If that path is congruent with our own, if the vital force of the remedy speaks to our own, then healing takes place.

This might well explain what happens when a patient takes the wrong remedy. When they are given a dose of a remedy that is not similar in action to the symptoms created by their own vital force. (And, remember, that as the symptoms expressed by each and every one of us are responses to our environment, they are created by our own vital force, our own life energy. Only when a person dies, when the vital force is extinguished, does this reactive mechanism responsible for the creation of symptoms stop functioning. And as the vital force within each of us is invisible and intangible, it must be noted that all symptoms are the product of our "energy selves," our invisible nature. This is why homeopaths believe that all healing therefore must also take place within the invisible and intangible parts of ourselves, in order for the physical bodies to follow in the ceasing of symptoms just as they do in their creation.)

When a patient takes the wrong remedy, nothing happens. The strategy within the remedy could not communicate with the patient. So nothing at all happens. The patient does not get any better or any worse. They do not feel energized or sleepy.

You most certainly cannot say the same thing about allopathic drugs. For better or worse, they always create a change. This change may soothe the patient or create utter havoc in their system. This gives the allopath a far greater opportunity for causing actual harm to his patient, as an ill-chosen medicine can have terrible results.

In homeopathic medicine, a single dose of the wrong remedy will do nothing. If this medicine is repeated again and again, however, the power of the remedy will ultimately be revealed through what is called a *proving*.

In a proving, a remedy is given repeatedly to the same patient, either through the utter ignorance of the homeopath, or in an attempt in a clinical setting, to establish the exact and complete medicinal action of a remedy. But whether the remedy is given to purposefully create a proving or not, the outcome is the same. The artificial disease state created by that remedy's action will become grafted upon that patient's system for as long as the remedy is given.

This last bit is important, because it again gives witness to my theory of what happens in homeopathic treatment. Even when a proving happens, when the power of the vital force of the remedy literally overwhelms the patient's vital force and they begin to "enact" the remedy, which is to say take on the physical, mental, and emotional symptoms of the remedy state, that grafted state can only stay in place for as long as it is renewed by a new dose of the remedy itself. When the last dose causing the proving has been given, the power of the remedy will begin to fade as the power of that dose comes to an end. And, when that has faded, the patient will be as he was before.

Even when a wrong, or dissimilar, remedy is given repeatedly, it cannot make any real or permanent change in the patient, because the vital force of the remedy and the vital force of the patient still cannot communicate. Only by a true similarity of the vital forces of patient and remedy can a change be made.

This does suggest that, in homeopathic medicine, there may well be varying degrees of similarity. That there might be more than one remedy that is potentially helpful for an individual patient. And that these different remedies may, in that they are more or less similar to the patient and his symptoms, be more or less effective in treating that patient.

And this is all true. This is part of what makes homeopathic medicine so damned difficult to practice. For each individual patient, there will be at least a handful of remedies that would do some good, that would speak to at least some of his symptoms. It is the job of the homeopathic physician to locate the best remedy, the one that is most similar in its action to the patient's own symptoms. This is the remedy that will work most effectively and be most permanent in its actions.

Each homeopath in each individual case is seeking what is called the *simillimum*, which is the correct or most similar remedy given in the right potency and the right number of doses. As we will see in future chapters, finding the actual simillimum is a very difficult task indeed. I believe that it is actually found in only very few cases. Most cases treated homeopathically are completed through the use of *similars* (also called *similes*), which are, in most cases, remedies that, while not perfect matches, still have enough in common with the case to be helpful. In some cases, the perfect remedy may well be found, but it is given in the wrong potency, or the wrong number of doses, thus upsetting the action of the simillimum. But as long as the degree of similarity is strong enough, healing can still take place. Because vital force is still communicating with vital force.

Homeopathy in Thought and Action

It was the American homeopath James Tyler Kent (1849–1916) who said that homeopathic remedies are homeopathic in two ways: by how they are made and by how they are used.*

Samuel Hahnemann systematized a method of working with medicines that was at once efficacious and benign. And along with this, he established a method of potentization that was and is incorruptible if followed precisely, giving practitioners and patients alike a sense of safety when using the medicines.

But these practitioners and, especially, these patients can only swallow the remedies with a feeling of total security when the use of remedies matches their creation.

In other words, you can take the best-made remedies—potentized perfectly from their source material—and bastardize them into something other than homeopathic by using them incorrectly.

Therefore, whether your personal goal is to be a wise practitioner or consumer of homeopathic medicine, it is important that you understand the methods by which these remedies are appropriately used, and the consequences of acting inappropriately.

Now that we've dealt with homeopathic thought, the philosophy that guides the practice of homeopathy, it is time to look at the practice itself. We will do so in the next few chapters.

---

* I think it was the American homeopath James Tyler Kent who first made this point, but I can't locate the exact quote. I add this footnote, therefore, so as not to deny his authorship, if he did indeed originate this statement. But whoever was the first to say it—it may have actually been me, and I've just forgotten when—it is true.

CHAPTER SEVEN

Playing by the Rules— Similars

T his should be the shortest chapter in this book.

This is because the Law of Similars is the one complete absolute in homeopathic medicine. While the Laws of Minimum and Simplex, under extreme circumstances may have to be bent or broken—a patient who has been in a car accident may well have to be given more than one remedy because there simply may not be time to wait and see the changes each remedy creates—the Law of Similars is always to be followed. Always. Without exception.

The Law of Similars states "likes may be cured by likes." Simplified, it is most often stated as "like cures like." In Latin, it is stated "similia similibus curantur." But the Latin is always listed in all the books on homeopathy. But in order to be a little more complete, and to try to drive the point home, I have tried to get translations into other languages as well:

- In French, they say "Les semblables guerissent les semblables."

- In German, it is "Gleichheilungen mogen."

- In Spanish, it is "Las guraciones del gusto teinen gusto."

- In Italian, it is "Le cure di simile grandiscono."

- In Portuguese, it is "As curas do gusto gostam."

- In Dutch, it is "Het lijkende met het gelijkende genezen."

- In Bulgarian, it is "Podobnoto se lekuva s podobno."

- In Polish, it is "Similia simily—bus curantur."

- In Turkish, it is "Okhshaar okshiyaani tokhtaadaar."

- In Japanese, it is "Onaji yoo na mono ga naosu."

- In Iran, it is "Moshaabeh moshaabeh raa darmaan mikonad" when translated into Farsi.

- Finally, it is "Sawa na sawa" in Swahili.*

The language changes, but the point remains the same: like cures like.

This is the principle that makes homeopathy homeopathic. Unless you work with the patient's symptoms, unless you give a medicine that, in a totally well person, would actually produce the same symptoms that the patient is experiencing, then you are not using homeopathic medicine.

Given all of Hahnemann's work and writings, given two hundred years of clinical evidence of the efficacy of homeopathic medicine, this should go without saying. And yet, again and again, I find that it *needs* saying. Consumers, students, and practitioners of homeopathy alike seem all too often willing to put their time and energy into finding rationalizations as to why they can ignore this simple fact instead of putting that same energy into a better understanding of homeopathy in its appropriate practice.

You cannot in any way and to any degree change this overriding principle and still say that you are practicing homeopathy. The Law of Similars is immutable and absolute. The moment that it is broken, the practitioner ceases the practice of homeopathy. This does not necessarily mean that what that practitioner is doing will not be effective—that is not for me to judge—but it will not and cannot be anything that could be called homeopathic.

The Law of Similars is broken any time a homeopathic medicine is given based upon anything other than the totality of symptoms. Any time that the practitioner pretends that he can isolate a particular symptom or set of symptoms from the totality

> The Law of Similars is immutable and absolute. The moment that it is broken, the practitioner ceases the practice of homeopathy.

of symptoms that the patient is experiencing. That the patient is *living*. The homeopath must always consider all that the patient is experiencing in body, mind, and spirit. This is true in simple acute cases, like colds or mechanical injuries, and it is true

---

* I want to thank the members of Lyghtforce, an Internet gathering place for students and practitioners of homeopathy for the translations I received. Individually, I want to thank Didi Abha Ruchira, Bernard Kol, Nader Moradi, Katarzyna Wyrobiec, Carol Thompson, Ginny Wilken, and Christo Karaivanov for their help. They took the time to send me these translations.

If you are interested in finding out more about Lyghtforce, or any number of other groups and data on homeopathy, including downloads of whole books that are in public domain, visit Homeopathyhome.com. You will find a wealth on information there and a whole world of help. Please check the Resource Guide at the back of this book for more information.

in deep chronic cases as well. Just as it is easier in acute cases to see what has changed from the moment before the onset of illness to the time during illness when treatment is sought, it is also easier perhaps, in these acute cases, to pretend that we can ignore the particulars of the case at hand—the patient's symptoms in their totality—and just treat the acute condition instead.

After all, doesn't the very presence of the acute condition in and of itself suggest a handful of remedies that are tried and true for these cases and would most likely be those that would treat this case as well?

That sort of thinking seems so sensible on the surface. So very likely to be true. But it is only true if you wish to seek allopathic treatment. If you wish to ignore the Law of Similars.

The Law of Similars tells us that we can never treat a disease, but always must treat the patient with the disease. This may sound like splitting hairs, but the difference between a treatment based on a disease and a treatment based upon the reactions of the patient suffering from that disease are profound.

Each patient is, first and foremost, a unique individual, one who experiences his disease in a manner that is unique to him. Therefore, the eyes of the homeopath must always remain upon the patient, in his unique experience of life, and never upon his disease. To focus on the disease is to accept the allopathic notion that the disease diagnosis itself suggests a course of treatment in and of itself. For the homeopath, the disease diagnosis alone is and must be a pointless thing. The disease diagnosis merely names a particular clump of symptoms. It in no way reveals what this particular patient's experience of those symptoms might be. And it is in that patient's particulars—the details of how he and he alone is experiencing the disease state—that the treatment can be found.

The remedy must be found that could create those same symptoms in a well person. Only that remedy will be totally effective in *expressing* those symptoms, in bringing them forth from the patient's body, leaving him in a state of health.

The whole point of homeopathic treatment is that the patient's symptoms are expressed, never suppressed. Therefore the patient with a cold will have to work through his cold. To suppress the symptoms of a cold is to drive the disease deeper into the body, and, in doing so, make the whole of his being a little weaker, a little more prone to disease.

When you have a cold and you take an allopathic medicine, you will for a time, lose the symptoms of the cold. But, as the impact of the medicine fades, those symptoms will reappear. The medicine has in no way affected the fact that you have a cold.

In the same way, a broken bone that is set has not in any way been cured. The person who puts the cast on the bone is counting on your body itself to heal itself and is only supporting the bone while it heals.

The patient with a broken bone who receives homeopathic treatment for that injury on the other hand, who takes a remedy like Symphytum, if it is appropriate to the individual case, is taking a medication that will actually help speed the healing process itself. That will leave the bone in better shape than it was before.

But you can only create this process of *expression*, wherein the patient moves through his illness more quickly than he would without treatment, and wherein he will likely experience his illness to a far lesser degree of discomfort than he would without homeopathic treatment, by staying true to the Law of Similars.

The moment that it is in any way bastardized is the moment in which the treatment ceases to be homeopathic in nature. Remember, as Kent said, homeopathic medicines are homeopathic in two ways—by how they are made and how they are used. And, in order for supposed homeopathic treatment to be homeopathic in impact, the practitioner must stay true to both parts. You have to use a remedy that has been fully and correctly potentized. And you have to use that remedy in a manner that is congruent with homeopathic philosophy, which is to say with the Law of Similars.

Homeopathy is truly holistic medicine. Homeopathy, and, most especially, the Law of Similars is all about *wholeness. Totality.*

It's all about the whole being—in body, mind, and spirit. You cannot touch, impact upon or isolate any part of the whole without affecting the whole. To pretend in any way that you have the ability to direct, restrict, or control a remedy in its impact upon the patient's body is to dream the allopath's dream. And it is to deny the truth that homeopathy reveals to us each and every time a homeopathic remedy works so miraculously when it is well chosen and well used.

This is not to say that every homeopathic remedy shares the same range of action. No, there are remedies that are deep in their action, that touch the very core of being, and there are remedies that are rather shallow in their action as well. There are remedies that will quite literally impact upon every cell of the patient's body and every aspect of his being and there are remedies that have a narrow range of action. There are remedies that work quickly and those that take a long time to create a change. But every remedy must be considered in its full range of action, however wide or narrow, deep, or shallow that may be. And every patient must be considered in the totality of his symptoms. And then the two—the remedy's actions and the patient's totality of symptoms—must be fully considered and matched.

This is how homeopathy is practiced. Nothing else can correctly be termed "homeopathic."

The Curmudgeon's Medicine

When homeopathy came to the United States, it was treated like every person, every food, every fashion that came from some other place to these shores, it was Americanized. Just like the award-winning foreign film or novel that is remade as an American movie, homeopathy has been "punched up" for American consumption. It has been made sexier. What is a cheap and effective medicine for millions of people in India, who daily stand in long lines to be quickly examined by a homeopath has become a luxury item in the United States, one that often involves skylights, potted palms, and incense. And that always involves the wearing of earth tones.

This Americanization of homeopathy (perhaps I should refer to it as the "capitalization" of homeopathy) has brought it dangerously close to its allopathic counterpart. The fact that remedies are now routinely sold in combination and mixed potency doses (which implies, of course, that if one homeopathic remedy or potency is good, then more than one should be even better, and, in the implication, manage to break all Three Laws of Cure simultaneously, which is no small feat) shows that the profit motive has warped homeopathy in much the same way that it has warped nearly everything else in our lives.

And so many rationalizations are given as to why these "improvements" of homeopathy have been made. My favorite is the one that insists that Hahnemann himself would be selling combination remedies (no doubt from his self-named chain of homeopathic pharmacies) or prescribing remedies in the treatment of disease were he alive today. This logic presupposes that Hahnemann would have turned his back on something that it took him a lifetime to perfect. And it is ludicrous. The fact that the people making such a statement are thereby placing themselves in a position to know what Hahnemann was thinking at the moment of his death and beyond is truly maddening.

There are also those who argue that, because of our increasingly polluted environment, we now must have more and stronger remedies. That the remedies made two hundred years ago simply will not do in our new technological age. The fact that Natrum Muriaticum, a remedy taken from simple table salt, can still work miracles, if you actually know how and when to use it, seems to escape them.

Oh, there are so many other arguments. So many reasons given by those who, in my opinion, are lacking in a true understanding of homeopathy, why they shouldn't have to actually learn it well enough to use it correctly before they begin their practice of homeopathy. Or begin selling a line of remedies.

For me, aged curmudgeon that I am—all bald and squinty—the most insulting thing is when those who think as I do, who actually don't see any reason to fix homeopathy when it is not broken, are referred to by the term "classical homeopaths." It is as if homeopathy were being lumped in with any other form of commodity, from Coca Cola onward, and that old farts like me are being relegated to still liking the original formula, while the new, young, hip folk all know that those Laws of Cure are just meant as a guideline, sort of like a curfew.

> Those words were *homios,* which means "similar" and *pathos,* which means "suffering." The term "homeopathy" therefore means "similar suffering" and contains the principle of the Law of Similars in the term itself.

Let's be very clear. There is no such thing as "classical" homeopathy, or "modern" homeopathy, or vanilla or lime homeopathy for that matter. This camp has only two divisions: homeopathy and non-homeopathy (allopathy and everything else).

Here we've dealt with the Law of Similars. Next we will look at Simplex and Minimum. Through the understanding of and appropriate use of these three principles, medicine becomes homeopathic (provided, of course, that said medicine was also correctly potentized). No other way.

Cling to the very term "homeopathy." When Hahnemann finally got around to naming his new system of medicine, one that in every way flew in the face of what was considered appropriate medical treatment in his day, he took two Greek words and blended them into one. Those words were *homios,* which mean "similar" and *pathos,* which means "suffering." The term "homeopathy" therefore means "similar suffering" and contains the principle of the Law of Similars in the term itself.*

Do you think for a moment that Samuel Hahnemann would have named his new medical art for a specific principle if he didn't consider that particular principle somewhat important to that new medical art?

Only by staying true to the Law of Similars can one ever be sure that they are practicing homeopathy, there's just no way around it.

---

* Hahnemann also coined the term "allopathy," which he took from the Greek *allos,* which means "different" and added it to pathos. I have always found it somewhat ironic that those who rejected Hahnemann's whole philosophy of medicine were still willing to accept his term for their own practice.

CHAPTER EIGHT

Playing by the Rules— Simplex

The Law of Simplex is, like Similars, very easily stated and easily understood. Unfortunately, even more than the Law of Similars, the Law of Simplex is somewhat fragile and easily broken.

Simplex simply tells us that we are to use one remedy at a time. And, in doing so, it forbids what Samuel Hahnemann called *polypharmacy*.

Polypharmacy

Simply put, polypharmacy is the practice of using more than one medicine at a time. This practice can apply either to allopathic or homeopathic medicine. In either case, it is an equally risky proposition.

When students of homeopathy first read Hahnemann's own theories as he presents them in the *Organon of Medicine,* they are often surprised that the first section of the book hardly references homeopathy at all. Instead, it deals with the practice of medicine in general, whether that practice is homeopathic or allopathic in nature. And one of the practices that Hahnemann rails against most strongly is polypharmacy.

The reason why should be fairly obvious, but perhaps it bears consideration. After all, the overabundance of combination homeopathic remedies on the shelves of our health-food stores gives us some indication that someone somewhere doesn't understand the problems created by the practice of polypharmacy.

As has been stressed again and again in these pages, medicine—allopathic or homeopathic—does not have one simple impact upon the human system. Any medicine has an entire sphere of action. Even the most benign medication will cause not just a single change, but will instead cause a number of changes to take place. Some of these will be common and expected. Others might well be quite surprising.

On the occasions in which the changes are surprising, even unsettling, the physician—again, either homeopathic or allopathic—will tend to say things like "Most people are not as sensitive to this medication as you are." And then they usually make a quick change in medication.

The reality remains that no doctor can predict exactly what any single medicine will do in the totality of its action until they have given the medicine to the patient. And even if the medication turns out to be tolerable for the patient—in other words, the good that it is doing outweighs the bad "side effect"—the doctor may well have to wrestle with dosage before things are brought into balance. How many times has an allopathic doctor had to try the same medicine in a more powerful or less powerful dose before the patient feels better? How often do doctors have to substitute one medicine for another before the patient can tolerate his or her treatment?

These are, of course, very common problems. Even in homeopathic medicine, after the case has been well taken and researched, it is more common than I would like to admit that the patient is given what seems to be a well-selected remedy and that remedy utterly fails to work. Or does not work in the manner in which it was predicted it would.

This is, of course, because prescribing medication involves a certain amount of playing the odds. Trial and error. The allopathic doctor will tend to give a medicine from the group of medications that are known to be effective for the disease that he is treating. Using his own clinical experience, he will choose the medication that has either given him the best response in the past, or that seems indicated by the patient's own characteristics—age, gender, general state of health, and so on.

Even the homeopath, after all that case taking and research, may find himself faced with a handful of remedies that could each arguably be helpful to the patient. And since that homeopath cannot know exactly what changes each remedy may bring about—what aggravations may arise, for instance—even he is, quite often, making his best guess as to what to prescribe, based upon his own clinical experience.

Indeed, in large part, that is what we pay doctors for—their clinical experience. We trust that, when we bring our ailments to them, they will first know what it is we are suffering from, and, second, what they can do to bring us back to a state of health.

But, in reality, we are asking them to know the unknowable. There is no way for anyone to ever know exactly what will happen when a medicine is given. In the same way, there is no way of "untreating" what has already been treated.

If every medicine is medicinal in its action, if it in some way acts as a catalyst to change in our bodies—change for better or worse—and if no one can know exactly what any given medicine will do in the totality of its action in any given case, then there is some risk involved in the use of any medication. Now, this risk is to a greater or lesser degree, to be sure. For instance, our government designates drugs that are available over the counter and drugs that are available by a doctor's prescription only. This is because the over-the-counter drugs are supposedly more or less benign, although history should show us that this is in all actuality not the case, as anyone with hypertension who takes over-the-counter cold or allergy medication can find out to their peril.

And that's the whole issue here—peril. The Three Laws of Cure in general and the Law of Simplex specifically have been put in place to make the practice of homeopathic medicine as safe as it can be. And, in all truth, I do believe that, if all three laws are followed to the letter, that homeopathic treatments are not capable of harming a patient.

If we cannot predict what a medicine will do, and if we cannot untreat what has already been treated (once a medicine has been taken by the patient, for better or worse, it has had some sort of impact) then doesn't it seem prudent that, when we give medication, we give it wisely and carefully?

We have certainly seen, in our recent history, the impact of giving antibiotics like candy. Over the past few years, the allopath's over-reliance on antibiotics has lead to weaker immune systems in their patients, who seem ever more vulnerable to infection, and to stronger and stronger strains of bacteria, that are ever more resistant to the antibiotics that used to kill them.

But what we refuse to see, in both allopathic medicine and in some foolish, bastardized forms of "homeopathic" medicine, is the danger of giving too many medications at one time.

It should be obvious why this is dangerous. If a doctor cannot predict what a single medicine will exactly do—whether it will be a helpful or harmful thing—before he gives it, then how the hell is he supposed to know what two, three, or four medicines will do if he gives them all at the same time? And how is he supposed to single out what medicine one is doing, as opposed to what medicines two, three and four are doing? If the patient reacts badly, how is he supposed to know which of the four medicines to adjust or change completely?

> If we cannot predict what a medicine will do, and if we cannot untreat what has already been treated . . . then doesn't it seem prudent that, when we give medication, we give it wisely and carefully?

This is what the practice of polypharmacy does: it creates a case that is such a muddle of information, of old symptoms getting better, perhaps, while new ones appear, or old symptoms simply changing, getting no better or worse, while new ones crop up, that the patient, over time, will no longer be curable. And polypharmacy will create this same muddle whether that medication is allopathic or homeopathic.

Surely in medicine, we ought to move wisely, stick with what we can know and trace and watch. And this means that we have to give fewer (one being best) medications and choose those medications more wisely, so that we as patients can actually get healthier as a result of treatment.

We have to quit breaking the Law of Simplex.

Compound and Combination Remedies

It occurs to me that, before I go further, I should perhaps give some indication of what exactly a combination remedy is.

It is exactly what it sounds like—one single pellet of medication that has been potentized with several different remedies. So that the patient, in letting that pellet dissolve on his or her tongue, is not just taking one remedy, but several at one time.

The chief problem with this—besides the fact that even by existing at all, these combination remedies are a form of polypharmacy and break the Law of Simplex—has to do with the proving of remedies.

As I have said earlier, homeopathic remedies are unique in the medical world because their action is proven on healthy humans. Homeopaths never use any form of animal testing in developing new medicines. Instead, the multiple actions of the remedy are uncovered in a double-blind study in which a group of healthy people take the remedy for a set period of time and record all the changes that occur while taking the remedy. The changes that occur most commonly become the changes that are most expected in the use of that remedy, although all are noted and considered in the selection of that remedy.

This whole process is called *proving*. If you remember, I earlier used the same term for the situation created when an incorrectly chosen remedy is given in repeated doses. I use the same term for both because both circumstances refer to exactly the same thing.

The remedy that is incorrectly selected (in that it is lacking in basic similarity with the patient's system) and repeatedly given will, as the doses mount up, create the symptoms associated with that remedy, as the remedy's potency temporarily overwhelms the patient's own vital force. In clinical provings, the same outcome occurs when healthy patients are selected and then are given repeated doses of a remedy in order to test what the actions of that remedy are.

The problem with combination remedies is that they tend not to be proven in their combined form. Instead, pharmacies take established and well-proven remedies and combine them in their already potentized state. This makes for something of a Frankenstein remedy, with Arsenicum's left leg, Lachesis's chest, Phosphorus' eyes, and so on. Because the combination has not been thoroughly tested *in combination*, there is just no way of knowing what it will do.

Along the same line, if you give a combination remedy that contains, among a dozen or so remedies, the one that the patient needs, then all is well—at least at first.

Say you are giving a combination remedy for allergies. With the first couple of doses, the patient feels much better. His allergies are relieved and his vital force is stoked. He feels good.

But, as each dose wears off, he takes another. And another. Over time, not only do his allergies return, but also he takes on new symptoms that hadn't bothered him before. Now his eyes are watering, in addition to his old post-nasal drip. Finally, disgusted, he stops taking the remedy altogether, and remains puzzled as to why it worked so well, but then stopped working.

The reason was simple. The remedy that he actually needed, that was actually similar in action to his own symptoms, worked perfectly. It relieved his symptoms. And had he been taking that remedy alone, his case would have been moving toward cure.

But he was taking that remedy as only one of a dozen remedies. And, as he took dose after dose, he began to prove the other eleven remedies, while the needed remedy continued to work toward cure. Now if you have eleven unneeded remedies that are beginning to prove themselves, and only one needed remedy that is doing all it can to move the patient to cure, which do you think is going to win? That's why the patient will begin to get some new symptoms. They are not new allergies, they are the signs of proving. And they are, in my opinion, reason enough not to mess with combination remedies.

Finally, please note that combination remedies should never be confused with *compound* remedies.

Compound remedies are those that combine more than one substance in the actual creation of the remedy. With compound remedies, the combining occurs while the remedy is still in the material state. It is then potentized in the usual way and then tested and fully proven as a single homeopathic remedy.

Examples of compound remedies would be Magnesia Phosphorica, which combines the substances magnesium and phosphorus into a single potentized remedy, or Calcarea Phosphorica, which combines calcium and phosphorus in the same way.

Compound remedies, because the actual substances are combined *before* potentization takes place and because they have been fully proven as homeopathic remedies, are an appropriate part of the homeopathic pharmacy.

Breaking Simplex

First, let's try to agree that no one practicing homeopathy either professionally or at home, is doing so in order to harm anyone. It is to be hoped that everyone who uses the remedies does so in order to bring about a cure.

But that does not mean that you can do no harm with homeopathic medicines.

To begin with, there are many "if onlys" in homeopathic case taking and case management. So many times when you are kept up nights wrestling with a case, angry at yourself that you can't see the remedy for the situation at hand. Certainly, there are the moments of victory, when you see the patient's eyes clear as the remedy dissolves in their mouth, when you see the aspect of pain leave their face, and a gentle sleep takes them over, from which they awaken refreshed and renewed.

But there are moments of terrible defeat as well. When what seems to be the best indicated remedy just does no good and the patient suffers. If that patient is someone you love, it can be a terrible, terrible thing, to be so helpless in the face of suffering.

This so often will lead us to make mistakes. It happens all the time in household prescribing.

Your child awakens in the middle of the night with a terrible earache. You suspect otitis media and you start looking for a remedy. You are a bit groggy from being awakened and certainly terribly concerned. Perhaps you are balancing your child against your chest and holding on with your chin as your try to look through your home guides to get some idea of a remedy.

Perhaps you give Pulsatilla 30C as your best guess. And you hold your child or rock him in on your lap in a rocking chair. Nothing happens. In a few minutes, you give another dose and wait again. Again, nothing. You try a third dose about a half hour later. Nothing. Frustrated, worried, and even more tired than before because it is about 2:00 a.m. by now, you get out the book again and select Silicea. You would do the 30C, but all you have is 12C, so you give that. Nothing happens.

By dawn, you have given a few more remedies. What you had on hand that the book mentioned. Those that you didn't have on hand, you just had to forget about, even if they sounded as good or better than the ones you used.

By morning, your child seems sicker and sicker. And nothing has worked. In the end, you feel like throwing all your remedies away and saying, "This crap doesn't work," and going back to the pediatrician for an antibiotic. At least you know that will work. (On this particular ear infection, anyway.)

In this case, out of love and concern, you have made quite a mess of things. You have given multiple doses of some remedies and many different remedies in a short time span. And each dose has done something. And all those somethings add up to an inability for any remedy to be able to do its job well. Too much medication, given in too low, or, especially, too high a potency can create such havoc that the patient may, in the end, just have to endure

> Simplex . . . forces us, when we take on the role of the physician, to think clearly and to treat wisely. And to only give a medication when we have a clear indication of what medication to give. And then only a single medication at a time.

the disease, at least from the standpoint of homeopathic medicine. As we will see in the next chapter, more cases are ruined by doing too much then by doing too little.

That's why Simplex is so important. It forces us, when we take on the role of the physician, to think clearly and to treat wisely. And to only give a medication when we have a clear indication of what medication to give. And then only a single medication at a time.

One at a Time

Now, what we mean by "one at a time" can differ dramatically from case to case. It depends upon the circumstances of the individual case and the nature of the case itself.

Certainly, for instance, in a true acute emergency, such as a simple but very traumatic mechanical injury, as might result from a car accident, you may well have to give different remedies much more closely timed together than you ordinarily would. And in the simple *acutes* (acute emergencies) that you find in the home, most especially when they happen, as they usually do, late at night and you have to make the most of your resources at hand, you may have to move from the first choice remedy to the second choice more swiftly than you might otherwise do. But the point remains the same: start with a single dose of a single remedy and give it an appropriate amount of time for the purposes of creating a curative response.

In an acute situation, that amount of time may be as short as five minutes. In a constitutional case involving chronic conditions, that appropriate period may be as long as a month. It depends upon the patient and the situation. But it always starts the same way: one remedy, one dose. (And if, as a lay practitioner, you have reached the second remedy and the second dose and no improvement has begun, then, in the best interests of the patient, it is time to call for help. Even if this means waiting for morning and soothing the patient as best you can, by making this decision and keeping records of exactly what you have done that didn't work, you still preserve the possibility that homeopathic treatment can bring about a cure in this case. If you keep trying different things, you may well spoil this case so that it cannot be homeopathically cured. As a final note, it is never my intention that we create homeopathic martyrs. If a case is beyond your help and no homeopath can be found, then by all means get the best allopathic care you can. Go to the hospital emergency room. The bottom line is that life should be preserved when it can. The consequences of allopathic treatment can be dealt with once the patient's life has been preserved.)

Rumplemeyer's

A few years ago, I attended a conference that a homeopathic organization sponsored at the St. Moritz Hotel in New York City.

I chose to take the train into the city because the keynote speaker of the conference was Dr. Edward C. Whitmont, who was then in the last years of his life. Whitmont was the author of two of my favorite books on homeopathy, *Psyche and Substance* and, especially, *The Alchemy of Healing*, both of which I strongly suggest that you read if you haven't already.

After what was an excellent lecture, Whitmont was brought back to the podium once more as part of the late morning question-and-answer period that was to fill in the hour before lunch.

I don't remember how it came up, but I do remember that this question-and-answer period became very heated on the subject of polypharmacy. And, as I remember it, it was an issue that split upon the generational divide. The older homeopaths, those who had labored in obscurity and, quite often, poverty throughout their careers, and who were still wearing very old suits, stood firm with the ideas that have come in recent years to be associated with what is called "classical" homeopathy. Which is to say, "actual" homeopathy, in that these practitioners stayed within the boundaries of homeopathic treatment as Hahnemann established them.

The younger practitioners tended to be those who were more or less willing to throw out the old rules and try new things. I especially remember one very prosperous-looking young practitioner who commented to the assembled panel that he had found in his practice that single remedies just did not work anymore. That patients now needed remedies in greater amounts and in combination to help them survive in our ever more polluted environment.

Whitmont, who had remained silent throughout the question-and-answer period, slowly reached out his hand and pulled the table mike to his mouth. He leaned in and said, quite simply, "Happily, that has not been my experience."

In saying so little he said so much. The young practitioner, who had neither been directly scolded nor in any way supported in the nonsense he was spouting, sat down, embarrassed.

Because everyone in the room knew exactly what Whitmont meant. Here was a man who dedicated his life to understanding homeopathy, to writing about it, and, above all, to practicing it. If he, in his wealth of experience had not faced the patient who needed multiple remedies in multiple doses, but, over all his years in practice had managed to cure his patients with a single remedy, then what did it say about this young practitioner, who needed to struggle so much more to achieve something resembling a cure?

After the question-and-answer period, I found that, to my great pleasure, I was invited to lunch with two very well-known homeopathic authors. One had written perhaps the definitive history of homeopathy. The other had written a very popular home guide that had helped revitalize interest in homeopathy in recent years.

As the old New York ice cream parlor, Rumplemeyer's was nearby, that's where we went.

The restaurant was filled to overflowing. Not only were there other folks from our conference present, but also there were nannies and their charges, children who were being rewarded for being good while their mothers shopped, and tourists by the tablefull.

After a short wait, we got a table in the middle of the restaurant, and gave our orders. While we waited for the food, we began to talk about each of their new books and about the day's events. It was in this way that we began to talk about the controversy that had been so stirred up that morning—whether the old rules of homeopathic practice still apply today as they did in Hahnemann's day.

Now, it would be hard for anyone other that a student of homeopathy to comprehend the passion of this discussion. Since no one but a student of homeopathy would have a clue as to what we were fighting about, much less really care at all whether or not a combination remedy is used.

But we were very passionate. As the older author sat with an expression on his face that was a mixture of amusement and embarrassment, the younger author (he's actually older than I, but a good deal younger than the other guy) and I got louder and louder.

Now, I don't know whether or not the fact that the younger author sells combination remedies from his company had anything to do with this espoused philosophy or not, but he stated quite clearly that not only was there nothing wrong with using combination remedies, but also that they were quite necessary.

He then brought up the subject of sports medicine, which had been the subject of his most recently published book. And he said that in many cases of sports injury, one remedy alone would not do the trick—that a combination of remedies was needed to achieve a cure.

I remember that my jaw just dropped at that point. After all, I had read this guy's books when I was back in Texas and taking my first homeopathic remedy that I had bought at the world's worst health-food store. Through his published works, he had been my first teacher.

For one of the very few times in my life that it has happened, I was rendered speechless. I just couldn't think of anything to say. Here he was literally the author of a book on sports medicine and was using that fact in order to give ballast to his theories. And, as I had not yet been published at all at that point, I chose to say nothing.

Instead, I ate my pickle.

For all these years, that moment has haunted me. We all have, in our lives, our own list of moments in which we did not speak, and another list of the things we should have said, but didn't. And this is one of mine.

I should have reminded the guy that he was insisting that he could know the unknowable. That once a treatment had been committed to, either with a single or a combination remedy, that there is no way to know what would have happened, for better or worse, if another treatment had instead been given. And that, while it may be possible to change the course of treatment as needed with good result, there are no guarantees, once a treatment has been given, that you can ever get back to the original window of opportunity—to the original circumstance of treatment. Any action taken can change the basic premise of treatment. Sometimes permanently, sometimes only temporarily. And since the patient is also going on with his life, changing and growing, there may never be a way back to the original circumstances that originally required treatment.

So to say that a combination of remedies will be needed is like saying that Arnica is the remedy for bruises. Such a statement insists that knowledge is held that simply can't be known. It sets up the illusion of control and the false hopes that are the heart of allopathy.

Can I, on the other side of this equation, know that the single remedy will do the full work? No. Might another remedy in that combination remedy be needed? Yes. Might all the remedies in that combination, at one point or another, be needed? Yes. But even if more than one remedy is ultimately needed in curing a case, the only way that we can treat safely and effectively is to treat with one remedy at a time.

After all, if one medicine, given in the right number of doses and in the right potency, can clear away all the symptoms associated with the patient's discomfort and restore him to health, why would you ever want to give more than one medication?

It is always and forever the role of the physician to do just enough to encourage the patient's own healing mechanism to make him well. Perhaps it has been a part of the Americanization of homeopathy that is needed to be perceived as "new and improved" in order to be relevant to today's restless consumer. But, if in all reality, you can do so much with a simple microdose of a single remedy, why would you want to do more?

CHAPTER NINE

Playing by the Rules— Minimum

In this allopathic world, in which most people's memoirs would be well titled "Pills I Have Loved," the Law of Minimum suggests that physicians should walk with very small footprints. That they should never shove when it is only necessary for them to nudge. In other words, they should practice at all times by using the least amount of medicine necessary in order for their patients to get well.

In homeopathic medicine, the practitioner can accomplish this single task in two ways. First by giving their medicines in lowest possible effective potencies. And, second, by giving their medicines in the fewest possible number of effective doses. It is important to note that, for the homeopath to work by the Law of Minimum, he must accomplish both of these goals simultaneously. If either aspect of Minimum is followed while the other is broken, the case is spoiled and the cure—that which is rapid, gentle, and permanent—will not be achieved.

Minimum Potency

Both the concept of lowest effective potency and of lowest number of doses possible are, therefore, equally important.

Certainly it is always important that the physician choose a potency of medicine that is just *slightly* stronger than is the disease state itself. If the potency is too low, it will not have the ability to remove the disease symptoms. If the potency is too high, it will cause aggravations in the case that may cause the patient undue discomfort.

An *aggravation* is the temporary worsening of the patient's disease symptoms. It is caused by the primary action of the remedy itself. In that the remedy is chosen by its ability—in a healthy person—to create the symptoms that the patient is suffering, then it makes sense that, if the remedy given is too powerful, it will itself artificially create even stronger symptoms before, through the body's own reactive healing mechanism, those symptoms are expressed and removed from the body.

Aggravations, therefore, can sometimes be a source of minor irritation—the patient with a cold will have a sore throat that grows a bit worse before getting a whole lot better. But, in the case of a patient who is in a chronically weakened state, aggravations can be dangerous things. They should, whenever possible, be avoided. The wise practitioner can avoid them by carefully choosing from the many different potencies in which most remedies are potentized.

Some practitioners even come, in a strange way, to think of aggravations as good things. After all, they reason, if a single dose of a remedy can cause an aggravation, then that must have been the right remedy, right? And, this, of course is true. Remedies cannot be proven in a single dose. And if a single dose of the wrong remedy will create no change at all, then a single dose that creates a profound change—even one that may be perceived as a negative change—must be at least a similar remedy, if not the best of all possible remedies. Through this thinking some practitioners come to practice by virtue of aggravations. They use them as guideposts. They actually will see them as a sign of cure. And, in doing so, will create needless discomfort for their patients. And ignore one of the major precepts of homeopathic cure—that it always be gentle.

In reality, initial aggravations can be a good sign—but only in cases of acute illness. When a patient has an acute ailment and the symptoms of that illness are stirred up by the initial dose of that remedy, then the practitioner can be assured that those same symptoms will soon subside substantially. In some cases of acute illness, I do not even think that it is possible to treat it effectively without some sort of initial aggravation. The degree of the aggravation can, of course, be made greater or less by the better or more reckless choice of potency.

But, in cases of chronic illness of any sort, no aggravation should take place with the initial dose of a remedy. Hahnemann tells us that, in chronic cases, the aggravation should occur toward the end of treatment. It happens at the moment just before the patient is made totally well. The chronic—or constitutional—case should have no initial aggravation. In fact, in the smoothest and perhaps best treatments for chronic illness, the patient should feel nothing at all at first, nothing, at least, of a medicinal impact. They should never feel the dizziness or weakness that we associate with many allopathic medicines. Instead, the patient should just, in some way, feel *better*. This simple improvement should continue throughout the course of treatment, until there is a sudden stirring up of symptoms. The skilled homeopath knows that, with this sudden aggravation, the patient is showing signs that he will soon be made well.

That aggravation, the one that happens at the end of treatment, is the appropriate aggravation for a chronic case. The aggravation that happens at the beginning of treatment is, to me, a sign not that the remedy is correct, but that the practitioner does not know what he is doing.

Another thing to understand about aggravations is that they are brief events. As I said above, in acute cases, the aggravation should last only for a handful of hours. After this initial worsening of symptoms they should then grow dramatically better. If the patient, after the aggravation, grows better, or if the aggravation continues for a period of days or longer, then we are likely not dealing with an aggravation at all, but with a proving.

Minimum Dose

Provings are to the practitioners who don't know when to give the second dose or remedy—or, more important, when *not* to give the second dose—what aggravations are to the practitioners who don't know how to wisely select their potency.

If the initial power of a remedy is expressed in its potency, then its full glory as a healing agent is shown through its repetition. In that *every* remedy has the ability to prove itself whenever it is given in sufficient doses, it is easy to understand what I mean by this. The initial dose of a well-chosen remedy can be dramatic in its action. But that same well-chosen remedy, repeated when called for, can work miracles.

The appropriate number of the doses to begin with for the purposes of curing any case homeopathically is one. Always begin with a single dose and then wait. The amount of time that one would wait before giving the second dose depends upon a number of things.

It first depends upon the patient himself. And especially upon his reaction to the first dose. In that the human healing mechanism is reactive in nature, it is important to give a dose of what you think is a well-selected remedy and then give that remedy time to work. If the patient is basically healthy and is experiencing

> If the initial power of a remedy is expressed in its potency, then its full glory as a healing agent is shown through its repetition. . . . *Every* remedy has the ability to prove itself whenever it is given in sufficient doses.

an acute illness in what is, for the most part, a healthy life, then you may find a nearly instantaneous result. But if the patient has been ill for some time, and if his vital force is diminished by his ordeal, then the healing process may be slower, and the increments by which he becomes well may be smaller. (In these cases, it is important that the potency of each dose of medicine be as closely considered as is the administration of those doses, in that any aggravation or proving of a remedy could further weaken the patient and further diminish his vital force.)

In the same way, the expected impact of a given dose also has to do with the potency given. A remedy given in a 9X potency will most often not create as great a change—for the better or worse—as will a remedy given in, say a 200C potency. Therefore, the expectation of just what the remedy will do is as linked to the potency of the remedy as it is to the vital force of the patient.

It is also linked to the remedy itself. Each remedy has a particular sphere of action—parts of the body that it tends to impact more than others. The totality of the actions of any remedy is fully explored as it is clinically proven in its effectiveness. Each remedy also has is own peculiarities of action as well. Some are very quick-acting, others take longer to impact a case. If you are using a remedy, like Psorinum, for instance, which often takes eight days to fully act, and you are expecting a quick response, you are setting yourself and the patient up for defeat. The unique ways in which each homeopathic remedy acts must be taken fully into account in its use.

All three of these aspects of the case—the patient's vital force, the potency of the remedy and its peculiarities of action—must therefore be taken into account before the remedy is used. As will be dealt with in greater detail in future chapters, there may be, for instance, times in which a similar-actioned, vegetable-based remedy may be called for in a case that might become aggravated by an animal-based remedy.

Provings

As disruptive as aggravations may be, the overuse of remedies to the point of proving them may well be even more injurious to the patient and likely to ultimately undermine the possible cure.

Provings often come disguised as aggravations. But they are aggravations that seem never to end. And these sort of provings, which can fool both patient and practitioner into thinking—if they are foolish enough to use aggravations as a yardstick of cure—that they are working toward a cure, when they are, in reality, ruining their chances of ever successfully ending the case. Instead, they are risking the allopathic outcome of a case that cannot ultimately be cured, but only managed through years and years of continual treatment, which is not at all the same as the cure that Hahnemann promised us. In the same way that those who practice by way of aggravations have thrown out the gentle aspect of cure, those who practice by way of provings toss out any idea of permanence.

This is the problem that is created when the remedy is given, in opening up the case, more than once. If it is given once and an aggravation occurs, then you can know that the remedy is similar enough to the case that it has mirrored it and made the symptoms more intense. Left alone, the patient should soon experience a reduction of symptoms and then the case can be looked at again and the idea of a second dose of that remedy or the use of another remedy can be addressed.

If the selected remedy is given once and nothing happens at all, for better or worse, then either the remedy was given in a potency that was too low to get the job done, to create a needed change, or perhaps the remedy was simply wrong and something else is needed. But, again, the case can be moved forward, and decisions can be made as to what is appropriate to do next based upon the data of the original case taking and the result of the initial dose.

But, if more than one dose is given right from the beginning, if the patient is told, as altogether too many patients are, to take the remedy every three hours and call back in a couple of days, then, right from the start, it is quite impossible for the practitioner to know what is going on. If the symptoms immediately grow worse, most practitioners will just assume that they are looking at an aggravation, and will sit back and congratulate themselves thinking that they have located the right remedy first time out of the box.

But what if they are not looking at an aggravation at all? What if, due to the fact that the remedy was not initially given in a single dose, but in multiple doses, they are looking at a condition in which the repeated doses of the wrong remedy—one that is in all actuality not in similarity to the case at hand—have set in place an artificial disease that is, through the repetition of the dose, growing stronger than the original disease state? After all, if you are working with common symptoms, sore throats and the like, then there are dozens and dozens of remedies that can create those symptoms in a well person. And therefore, the patient who reports that his sore throat is getting worse may well be reporting a proving of the remedy and not the aggravation caused by a higher than needed potency of the right remedy.

Often, by the time that this practitioner figures out some days later that, indeed, they have created a proving and not an aggravation, they may have already muddled the case. After all, while, as I have said more than once, one dose of the wrong remedy will do nothing, repeated doses may well spark a long-term change. It may, after a proving, be quite impossible for the patient to get back to the place he was in before the onset of treatment for quite some time, if at all.

Simply put, practitioners who allow for provings in their patients through the overuse of remedies—well selected or not—spoil more cures than do any other practitioners. Worse, they not only ruin individual cases, but, if allowed to continue their overuse of the remedies over time will spoil that patient's ability to get well at all, at least through the use of homeopathic medicines. Time and again, I have seen patients who, through the overuse of homeopathic medicines, have become so muddled in their symptoms that there is no longer a way in which to get a handle on their case.

Knowing When to Stop

This brings up another important point—the fact that the case was ruined by the overuse of a homeopathic remedy does not always imply that the remedy used was the correct remedy. In fact, it could have been the absolutely best choice for a remedy and it could have been given in the correct potency. But, if you don't know when to not give the next dose of a remedy, you are going to ruin a lot of cases.

If a correctly chosen remedy is given, but given in more doses than are actually required in order to bring about a cure, then a proving will result. Think about it, a patient has a specific group of symptoms and a remedy is chosen based upon its ability to create in a healthy person the same symptoms that the patient is experiencing. If that remedy is given in a single dose and the action of that dose noted and then repeated as needed, the patient will, over time, become stronger and stronger in his vital force and his symptoms will be expressed and, ultimately, will cease to be.

That's how it's supposed to work. But what happens if you have a practitioner who, instead of judging each dose and monitoring it, just tells the patient to take the medicine three times a day—or once, or twice, or any other amount suggested by timing instead of actual need—and come back for a follow-up in a month? Well, if that patient is lucky, and the practitioner has not told them to take an amount of medicine that is beyond what is needed, the patient will return in a month feeling much better. But, if that practitioner has not correctly judged the case in his rubber stamp prescription, then the patient may, within the course of the month, become much sicker.

Say that patient needed only a single dose of the remedy to get the job done. This is unlikely in many cases, but it is likely that he will need a finite number of remedy doses. Instead of his actual need being the reason for the next dose, a set amount of time has been substituted. This implies that the practitioner can know precisely how long each dose of the medicine will be effective, which he most certainly cannot. It also implies that each dose of medicine will, in fact, be potent in the patient's system for the exact same amount of time, which is nonsense. While the practitioner is giving the patient a sense that he is all-knowing, he is, in all reality, practicing very sloppy homeopathy and risking the good health of his patient.

Just as every remedy has its particular sphere of action, each remedy has an arc of action as well. Some, like Aconite, work very quickly and for a relatively short amount of time. Remedies like this are naturally more geared in their action to acute situations. Other remedies, like Silicea, tend to work more slowly. Some of these will also work more deeply than do the quicker remedies, although this is not always the case. In the same way, some of these slower remedies tend to not bear repeating as well as do others.

The wise homeopath has studied well enough to know the arc of the action for the remedy he intends to give. And if he does not, he should surely look it up in his Materia Medica before giving it to the patient. Just as some remedies may be counterindicated for a given patient by their tendency to stir up aggravations, so, too may some remedies be counterindicated by the fact that they do not repeat well in any case, or because they cannot be repeated very often in a case that calls for quick movement forward.

At any rate, the arc of activity determines when the remedy should be repeated, if it is to be repeated at all. When a well-chosen remedy is given, the patient will undergo a change. That, after all, is the whole point of medicine, to elicit a change. When the remedy is well chosen, which is to say that the remedy itself is similar to the needs of the patient and the potency of the remedy is in balance with the patient's needs. The change created by the dose of this remedy may range from a deep, peaceful sleep, to a shifting or ending of symptoms, to a general sense of wellness—we will look more deeply at this phenomenon in future chapters—but the change will be objectively noticeable. Measurable. And as long as that improvement, that change, stays in place, there is simply no reason to give another dose of the remedy.

This is why it is so very foolish to give more than one dose of a medicine until you see what that medicine will do in the case at hand. If one dose will get the job done, why would you ever want to give two doses? With each new dose, you further engage the risk of pushing the case into a proving, and, in proving, you engage the risk of making changes in the patient's life that you do not want to take responsibility for making. Do as little as you have to do in order to get the job done—nothing more. Leave little footprints.

In leaving little footprints, it is only appropriate to give a second dose of medication when the arc of the first dose has begun its downward curve. Think of a literal arch, how it shoots up to the sky, curves softly and then falls dramatically to the ground. The action of the remedy will work in the same way. Now, some remedies have a more dramatic arc than do others, but all remedies in their actions will be like short stories, with a beginning, a middle and an end. If you give the second dose too soon, you cannot know the full action of the remedy, you fail to learn its impact upon the patient and what can be expected from it in terms of the complete cure. Further, you risk giving the remedy too often and proving it.

> In homeopathic treatment we always seek to give the mildest potency of remedy possible in the least number of effective doses in order to get the job done.

If you give the second dose too late, once the arc is slamming into the ground, you do not risk proving the remedy, but you make the patient's cure less gentle than it has to be. As the first dose begins to fade, the patient's improvement may begin to fade with it. You will see an increase in symptoms, a lowering in energy and wellness.

You don't want to give the second dose before you begin to see some signs that the first dose is fading. In this way, you are going to have to see a return of some symptoms, or a decrease in energy—again, something objectively measurable—before giving the remedy again. The well-timed second dose comes just as the first is beginning to fade, so that the arc of this remedy carries the patient's energy upward again with it, allowing them to retain the improvement that they had already begun and move forward to increased vitality.

Dosage and Potency

In learning to study the arc of the action of each dose of a medicine, a practitioner can learn something about potency as well. Remember the aspects of the Law of Minimum, potency and dosage, are intertwined. They will each support the other.

Therefore, if a patient is given a particular remedy in a particular potency, and if the arc of that remedy is much shorter or weaker than it should be, then the practitioner will have a strong indication that he has likely selected a pretty good remedy, but that a higher potency is needed to get the job done.

More on this ahead in case management, but, for now, remember the implications of the Law of Minimum. That neither the potency of the remedy selected, nor the number of the doses given should ever take what might have been a simple homeopathic cure and make it into a muddled mess. Long-term management of the "walking ill" is the domain of allopathic medicine. Rapid and gentle and permanent cure is the goal of homeopathic treatment.

Remember, even if homeopathic medicine, like allopathic medicine, involves giving pills, it is still the ultimate goal of homeopathic treatment that the patient should not have to take anything that may be called medicinal in order to be well. In homeopathic treatment we always seek to give the mildest potency of remedy possible in the least number of effective doses in order to get the job done. And, once the job is done, there is no further reason to medicate.

As with so many other aspects of life, we have to learn, in homeopathy, to leave well enough alone.

CHAPTER TEN

Inside Out and
Upside Down

Before any cases get taken and any remedies given, it is important that we have some sort of understanding as to how we get sick and how we move toward cure.

Perhaps our best guidelines for the healing process come from Constantin Hering, a German homeopath who had the excellent fortune to be born on January 1, 1800. In his eighty years of life, Hering started out training to be an allopathic doctor studying under the mentorship of a Dr. Robbi, who was himself a rather rabid opponent of all things homeopathic.

Because of Robbi's vociferous attacks on homeopathy, a publisher approached him to write a book on the subject. And because the young Constantin was Robbi's student assistant, he was assigned the task of helping Robbi with his research. Unfortunately for Robbi, Hering found much that he liked in the writings of Samuel Hahnemann.

When Hering contacted Hahnemann and let him know of his appreciation of homeopathy, Hahnemann—who had been all but driven out of Germany for his beliefs and could not support his family through the practice of medicine—advised the younger man to keep his mouth shut and to graduate from medical school and then practice medicine as he saw best. Instead, Hering spoke up, letting Robbi know of his change of thinking and then himself changed medical schools in order to get his medical degree.

Over time, Constantin Hering became one of the great practitioners of homeopathy, as well as one of the founding fathers of the homeopathic movement in the United States. In 1844, he became the founding president of the American Institute of Homeopathy.

Because of his belief that "the stronger the poison, the stronger the cure," he introduced the idea of using nitroglycerine as medication and proved the venom of the bushmaster snake as the homeopathic remedy Lachesis.

Without him, the practice of homeopathy in the United States would be a very different thing today. And, indeed, the practice of homeopathy worldwide would have been less for his absence.

With all that he accomplished in his lifetime, perhaps his most important contribution had to do with his observations on the homeopathic process of cure and how it generally takes place.

Hering's Law

In what is called Hering's Law* or "The Rule of Direction of Cure," the process of cure created through homeopathic treatment is described as being both orderly and capable of being reproduced from case to case.

Hering tells us that as the process of cure plays out, the patient's symptoms will improve from the top of his body downward, from more vital to less vital organs and from the most recent symptoms to the earliest symptoms.

Before going forward, let me note, in that Constantin Hering was in a way stating an absolute fact in putting forth his findings, it is perhaps an overstatement to call the observations a "law." It is, instead, a generalization that describes the usual flow of symptoms in successful homeopathic treatment. Which is to say that we ought not to cling to these observations as we would to the Three Laws of Cure. In no way should we panic if a homeopathic treatment does not precisely follow the pattern. Instead, it should be considered a useful method by which we can check our work and discern whether or not a particular case seems, in general, to be moving in the right direction.

Let's take it apart. First, Hering is telling us that, in his experience as a homeopath, when the patient is, as a whole being, moving from a state of disease to a state of well-being, that his symptoms will disappear from the top of this body downward. When you think about it, this first statement and the second—which tells us that symptoms will, in the process of cure, move from the more vital to the less vital parts of the body—are connected. As most of our "important" component parts tend to be contained in the top part of our bodies—the brain is, after all, in the head and the heart in the chest, just to name two—the patient will fulfill both the first and the second observation if his symptoms move from his head to his arms and legs, as the extremities, all things considered, must be called less important, if one is forced to make such a decision.

---

* Note that, while this description of the process of homeopathic cure is today known as "Hering's Law," Constantin Hering (1800–1880) never referred to it as such. He first described the process in 1845, in his preface to an edition of Samuel Hahnemann's own book, *Chronic Diseases*. But it was the American homeopath James Tyler Kent, who, upon reading the preface dubbed the observations "Hering's Law." As perhaps the most influential homeopathic educator of his day, Kent had the ear of a whole generation of American homeopaths, all of whom followed his lead in learning Hering's Law.

The process that moves the symptoms from the more vital to the less vital organs is one of expression. Just as the use of allopathic drugs weaken the overall vital force and suppress illness deeper into the body—which is to say, from less vital organs to more vital organs—an appropriate homeopathic treatment will express the same symptoms, allow the body to release them, and, in doing so, will continually move them closer and closer to the surface.

(Again, this is the total inverse of the ravages caused in allopathic medicine, in which hay fever treated with steroids can move deeper into food allergies, colitis and such, and then, with continued treatment, deeper still, into possible migraines. This was the pattern of allopathic suppression in my own case. And, through homeopathic treatment, the progression of the symptoms reversed, bringing the symptoms down-ward from the head, the migraines, to the digestive organs, and, finally to the nose and the skin in the form of seasonal allergies. And, in doing so, I know that that final jump from the stomach to the nose is a movement upward as well as outward and, therefore, presents a less than perfect example of Hering's Law. And this will quite often be the case, which is why I warned you that Hering's Law was just a guideline and not an absolute.)

For the purposes of observation, it should be noted that symptoms of the brain must be considered as being the most vital. Heart ailments are second, followed by symptoms of the endocrine system, the liver, and the lungs and kidneys. Symptoms in the bone are next. Muscle symptoms are next. And symptoms on the skin are the least important, as the skin is considered to be the least important organ of the body.

Again, to consider the inverse action of allopathic treatment, it should be noted that skin symptoms are very often those that, when suppressed, become the root sys-tem for any number of deep, chronic conditions. If we could simply observe in how many cases diaper rashes in babies are suppressed into ear infec-tions, which are then suppressed, with continued use of antibiotics, into be-havioral disorders and other deeper disease, then we might well be forced into admitting that Hering was on to something.

In Chapter 1 of this book, I wrote of the idea of some sort of rash being the first disease state, one that was so irritating that it elicited the first medical treatment in the form of that magic leaf. I purposely chose a rash because many homeopaths indeed believe that skin conditions

> . . . many homeopaths indeed believe that skin conditions were likely the first diseases, and that, through the suppression of these conditions, through the use of allopathic doses of plant-based remedies, these conditions were driven deeper and deeper, becoming the root system of the myriad diseases that now plague mankind.

were likely the first diseases, and that, through the suppression of these conditions, through the use of allopathic doses of plant-based remedies, these conditions were driven deeper and deeper, becoming the root system of myriad diseases that now plague mankind.

Whether or not this is actually true, we cannot know. But we can understand the principle of expression, by which, through skilled homeopathic treatment, disease symptoms move from the deepest level of the body to the outermost. Therefore, in many cases, most especially cases involving long-term treatment of chronic diseases, the patient will often notice a rash—perhaps a rash that they used to get as a child but haven't seen in many years—as the treatment is reaching its successful conclusion. If the patient and practitioner are wise enough to leave that rash alone, it will soon disappear and the patient will be well. If that rash is treated and driven back into the body, illness will continue.

Revisiting Illnesses Past

The rest of Hering's Law tells us that through homeopathic cure, the symptoms of illness will disappear in the opposite order in which they appeared. Therefore, the symptoms at hand, the ones that were troublesome enough to get the patient into the practitioner's office, will most often disappear rather quickly. Which is a good thing.

And if these symptoms are the sum total of the actual disease, then the patient will very quickly be made well. This is the case, of course, for some acute conditions. If the patient had a true acute condition, then, in removing these symptoms, the practitioner will be returning the patient to a state of health.

But, very often this is not the case. Most of us, unfortunately, have conditions that are more chronic in nature, and may involve a combination of past suppressive treatments, poor lifestyle choices, ongoing stress and strain, a polluted environment, and a flawed genetic makeup. This combination can make for a homeopathic treatment that involves more than one remedy, potency, and dose. It can involve an ongoing approach to treatment that requires multiple remedies—issued one at a time, of course, and only as needed, over a period of time—that requires great skill on the part of the practitioner and much patience on the part of the patient.

But it is in these cases that you can truly see the flow of symptoms as a cure is taking place. In cases in which patients have been ill for a long period of time, you will see the patient reliving his old illnesses as, one by one, the layers of suppression are cleared. This will, of course, tend to take place from the most recent to the most ancient symptoms.

Please note that, in revisiting the old symptoms, the patient will not have to suffer from the ailments as he has in the past. Instead, the "revisitations" will tend to be gentle things, the symptoms only an echo of the past. The patient may report to his

practitioner that he is having a bit of a skin condition that he has not had since ado-
lescence, or a ringing in his ears that he hasn't had in twenty years. The homeopath
who has taken an orderly case and managed it well will know to do nothing to treat
these symptoms, that they will soon fade.

But things are not always that simple.

And what is thought to be acute may sometimes be a good deal deeper and more
complex. In such a case, the patient who has been treated with a homeopathic remedy, instead of just getting better as expected, may seem to have been made a good
deal sicker by his remedy. Old symptoms may flare up again as the new symptoms,
those for which treatment was sought, disappear.

This is because not every *perceived* acute condition is truly an acute condition.
Often we tend, both in our own lives and in the lives of our loved ones, to fail to connect the dots as we should. For instance, the child who gets a cold a year and recovers
from it promptly and completely is likely to be getting a cold each year as his immune
system grows and learns. Nothing is wrong, everything is moving along and developing as it should.

But the child who gets three or four or more colds a year is often not suffering
from three or four different ailments a year, but, instead, is showing signs that there is
a deeper chronic condition at work. We'll go into this in more detail in the next chapter on the levels of treatment, but it is important to note here that Hering's Law is not
only a guideline into homeopathic treatment, but also, when considered in all its
implications, an insight into the nature of illness as well. It reveals to us not only how
we get well, but also how we move deeper and deeper into illness. How our illnesses—
mental, emotional, and physical, pile one on top of another in successive layers as,
instead of truly healing them and letting them go, we suppress them deeper and deeper and cling to them, to the point of building our lives around them. What matters,
therefore, is not the label of "acute" or "chronic," but the real nature of the disease
itself—where it has come from in its root cause, and how it has been suppressed again
and again, always into something deeper and more devastating to the vital force.

Disease moves ever deeper as it is suppressed. It moves from the extremities
deeper into the more vital organs, from the kidneys and lungs and liver into the heart
and brain. It moves, in doing so, from the outside in and the bottom upward. And, in
doing so, it layers itself, so that the oldest, and perhaps simplest symptoms (in terms of
homeopathic treatment) are buried below layer after layer of ever deeper and ever
more complex syndromes of symptoms.

Invisible Symptoms

In considering all these many layers of complex, intertwining ailments, we must
remember that not every symptom is one that can be measured and seen. Many of our

symptoms, indeed, our most important symptoms, are those that cannot be charted in any physical way.

But these invisible symptoms, those of the mind and the emotions, can have a profound impact.

They are, in fact, easily the equal of any physical symptom. And while some homeopaths would consider mental/emotional symptoms to be, as a whole, deeper and more important than the physicals, most, I think, would agree that mental and emotional symptoms run parallel to the physical and, like them, have a range of lesser and greater, more and less important symptoms. Therefore, the patient who exhibits the emotion of anger along with his physical aches and pains must have that anger listed along with and equal to any of those physical aches and pains. Homeopathy, remember, treats the whole man—body, mind, and emotions.

This is another philosophical component that separates homeopathy from allopathy. When was the last time that a doctor considered the fact that, during your cold, you felt very, very angry along with the stuffy nose, constipation, sore throat, and chills? The allopathic doctor might well note your anger, and perhaps hope that the next patient is a little easier to deal with than this one was. But the homeopath will use that anger as a guideline that, along with the other symptoms experienced, might well lead him to the remedy Nux Vomica. Just as a lack of anger in a case that otherwise suggested Nux might well counterindicate its use.

Just as the physical symptoms do, the emotional and mental symptoms will display a range of potency. Over time, a certain lack of concentration may deepen into disinterest, paranoia or a complete delirium. In the same way, an emotion as simple as anxiety may deepen into phobia or clinical depression. These invisible symptoms must be taken into account as clearly and thoughtfully as any physical symptoms in the initial case taking. And, once recorded they must be followed carefully as they, too move from more serious to less serious. And from the most recent symptoms back to the older, more engrained patterns.

In other words, to fully apply Hering's observations concerning the curative process of homeopathic treatment, you are going to have to keep your eyes on the whole patient as he moves from the constriction of illness to the relative freedom of health. And just as, in the selection of a remedy, it is necessary to consider the whole being of the patient in body, mind and emotions, it is important, in managing the case and following the curative process, that you continue to consider the whole. A patient who is growing

> The patient who, after treatment, sits before you with clear eyes and a clear mind, who moves to his chair with the freedom of movement that suggests a total freedom from pain, that is the patient who can be said to be well.

stronger in body but more phobic is not a patient who is undergoing a cure. In the same way, the patient who says that he is more able to understand himself and his motivations, and even able to forgive what to date he has been unable to forgive, but who is still beset with his physical complaints, is a patient who is certainly moving in a positive direction, but who has in no way completed his curative journey.

The patient who, after treatment, sits before you with clear eyes and a clear mind, who moves to his chair with the freedom of movement that suggests a total freedom from pain, that is the patient who can be said to be well.

CHAPTER ELEVEN

Susceptibility

On the subject of susceptibility, Hahnemann writes, "The—partly psychical and partly physical—inimical potencies in life on earth (which we call disease malignities) do not possess an absolute power to morbidly mistune the human condition. We become diseased by them only when our organism is just exactly and sufficiently disposed and laid open to be assailed by the cause of disease that is present, and to be altered in its condition, mistuned, and displaced into abnormal feelings and functions. Hence these inimical potencies do not make everyone sick every time."*

The Sources of Disease

Medically, we are taught that there are many causes for diseases: they can be the result of direct contact with a microorganism, or they can be toxins that have been inhaled, ingested, or are part of our environment.

Or they can be created through the use of allopathic medications of all sorts. In fact, new diseases created through medicating old diseases are fairly common in allopathic medicine. This is so common in modern allopathy that doctors have even coined a term for the diseases that they are creating by drugging their patients. They call them *iatrogenic conditions*. (I can't help but note here that, once again, standardized allopathic medicine has done something absolutely outrageous in creating new diseases by the dozens through the use of allopathic drugs, and they react, not by rethinking their treatments, but just by giving these mistakes a name and a category of medicine. In doing this, they continue the illusion of control by implying that, in naming this category of diseases, they are aware of them and are in control of the situ-

---

* The above is aphorism #31 of Hahnemann's *Organon*. In his own footnote to this aphorism, Hahnemann concludes that, in his description of disease above, he wished us to understand that diseases "are not mechanical or chemical alterations of the material substance of the organism; they are not dependent on material disease matter. They are solely spirit-like, dynamic mistunements of life."

ation. No doubt the allopathic solution to the poisoning of the patients with medicine is just additional medicine that is given to counter the symptoms created by the
original medicine. All of this implies that, had Dr. Frankenstein only thought to
name his monster, he would have been able to control the monster's actions.)

It should be noted that, in aphorism #74 of the *Organon*, Hahnemann states that
the diseases that are the result of violent allopathic treatment are themselves the
hardest to cure. In aphorism #75, he concludes, "I regret to say that when they have
been driven to some height, it seems to be impossible to invent or devise any curative
means for them."

In just as troublingly a manner, diseases can be created through use of vaccinations.

Just as the allopathic drugs that are given for one purpose, but in their multiple
actions create new and perhaps more violent symptoms, vaccinations, which are
given in the hope that they will allow the patient to ward off specific illnesses—block
susceptibility—can actually create circumstances of disease far worse than those they
are meant to forestall. In a condition known in homeopathic medicine as *vaccinosis*,
any number of chronic conditions, from allergies to asthma, rheumatoid arthritis, and
eczema can be artificially grafted to the patient through the administration of a vaccine.* This grafting of symptoms can lead to years, or even a lifetime, of needless
suffering.

Finally, we are also taught that emotional shock can be responsible for physical
disease, as can ongoing emotional stress. Giving us the psychologist's viewpoint,
homeopath Edward Whitmont taught that those things that cannot be absorbed on a
psychological level will manifest as physical illness.

The True Source of Disease

But whichever of these broad categories seems, in a particular case, to be the source of
a given disease, Hahnemann tells us, in aphorism #31, that the true cause, the under-
lying cause is always the same: that "they are solely spirit-like, dynamic mistunements
of life."

---

* It should be noted that the term vaccinosis is not from Hahnemann, but was coined by James
  Compton Burnett (1840–1901) at some point in the late 1890s. Like Hahnemann before
  him, Burnett was not against all vaccinations, and, in fact, held them in great interest. As
  Edward Jenner (1749–1823), the developer of the cowpox vaccine, and Hahnemann roughly
  were contemporaries, we can only guess the impact that Jenner had on Hahnemann's work.
  But surely vaccines were, at least at first, of some interest to homeopaths, in that they
  seemed to so clearly display the Law of Similars at work. Since vaccines made use of minute
  amounts of the very toxins that cause disease to build immunity to that same disease, they
  must have seemed like a good idea. What vaccines ignore, however, is the patient's own
  unique status and the very principle of susceptibility discussed here. Using a vaccine to treat
  two patients may leave one all the better for treatment while poisoning the other.

I love that phrase "dynamic mistunements of life."

It, of course, suggests perhaps the best reason for seeking homeopathic care above and beyond the allopathic. If we can accept the fact that all illness at its core is a disruption not of meat or chemicals, but of the spirit—the vital force that animates each of us and allows each of us to heal—then it can only follow logically that a medication that ignores the spirit (while, ironically, still counting on it ultimately for every healing in every case of disease) and reduces every aspect of our being to some sort of chemical reaction and then treats that reaction with yet another chemical simply cannot bring about a cure.

> If the true cause of disease is on the dynamic level, then only some form of medication that speaks to that level of being can bring a cure.

If the true cause of disease is on the dynamic level, then only some form of medication that speaks to that level of being can bring a cure.

While the topic of the spirit and the healing process will be the topic of Chapter 19 of this book, it should be noted here that, if you are going to narrow down your medical treatments to those that work on a dynamic as well as a physical level, then you have pretty much narrowed down to just two forms of treatment: homeopathy and acupuncture. In every other form of medicine, including herbal medicine, you are, as a patient, pretty much a bunch of chemical reactions that somehow makes the meat and bone that houses you get up and walk around. In that these treatments do not reach that "somehow" part of your being—that which animates the meat—they cannot reach deep enough into your being to really do much of anything.

Susceptibility and Disease

For an individual to become ill, something must disrupt or distort that patient's vital force. In that vital force is an active principle, something that is always in motion, always growing and learning, this disruption could well be in the form of a block. Anything that blocks the vital force, either from the point at which the energy force flows into the body, or at any point within the body, will result in illness.

This is a nice esoteric definition of illness and how it happens, but, unfortunately, it does not answer the question of exactly why we get ill. Why two people can experience the same "morbific" catalyst and only one will become ill. As I have said before, disease tends to follow the logic that allows me to bastardize Abraham Lincoln's truism into "disease can effectively attack some of the people all of the time and all of the people some of the time, but no disease can effectively attack all of the people all of the time." The reason for this has to do with the principle of susceptibility.

This principle tells us that, in order for some catalyst to cause the symptom-response within us to create a disease state, there has to be some common bond between that catalyst and ourselves. The nature of that bond determines the degree to which a given disease will be able to install itself with a greater or lesser number of humans. These catalysts can be highly specific in their action, and will, therefore only find a limited number of people who have a vulnerability to that catalyst. Or they can be more general in action, so that a high percentage of people who come into contact with the catalyst will experience disease symptoms as a response.

This is certainly true of new diseases. A new strain of influenza, for example, can become a global pandemic before the disease catalyst itself mutates in time into something less violent.

Epidemics are examples of disease catalysts that are the most general of all in their action. Not only are the infected individuals highly likely to experience disease symptoms, but those symptoms also will be very similar in case after case, individual after individual. And the symptoms will be easily transmitted from person to person.

Because of all this, epidemics are treated differently in homeopathic medicine than are outbreaks of other sorts of diseases.

Because of the speed with which an epidemic, or in our more modern situation— thanks in no small part to just how common global air travel has become—a pandemic moves, and because of the similarity of symptoms from case to case, and, finally, because the origin of all the cases involved in a pandemic are the same, a homeopath can consider all the individuals affected in the pandemic to be part of a single case. In true pandemics, all those suffering from the same condition may well be treated by a single remedy, with the potency and dosage adjusted to each patient's individual needs. Where homeopaths will most often put great effort and energy into determining the totalities of an individual case, in a time of pandemic, the emphasis must be placed upon the selection of a remedy whose action is in greatest similarity to the picture of the fast-spreading disease as it has commonly been experienced. If you will, a pandemic offers a picture of an acute ailment that can attack the human race as if it were a single entity, an individual.

This is the only instance that I know of in which such a practice of the homeopathic art is acceptable. And, certainly, by treating the group as if it were an individual, the treatment will not be as effective from individual to individual as a full case taking would allow. And some individuals will surely fair better than others from their treatments. But in the case of a pandemic, the circumstances, sadly, dictate the course of action.

So, the word "pandemic" describes a situation in which nearly every one of us will be reactive to a catalyst of disease. But, thankfully, this is a rather rare occurrence. More commonly, these catalysts will be held at bay, either through simple geography, or by other factors. Certainly the environment into which a catalyst is released will play an important part. The bacteria that is loosed into an area of filth, in which individuals drink unclean water, will have a far greater chance of taking hold and spreading than will the same bacteria let loose into a relatively sterile environment.

In the same way, an individual's lifestyle plays an important role in their sickness and health. The individual that eats a healthy diet, exercises appropriately, and avoids stress will find that he is ill far less often than is the individual whose lifestyle encourages disease.

But, as Hahnemann tells us, in the end, it comes down to vital force.

There are some of us who have very strong vital force. In whom there are no blocks, only free-flowing energy. These people may be said to be very healthy. As they go through their days, they, like all of us, come into contact with many different disease catalysts, as well as many other stressors, and yet they do not get sick. Their bodies do not react to the catalysts because none of them are strong enough to elicit a response. In the same way, none of the usual environmental stressors have the power to create a disease response. And the individual stays healthy.

> . . . as Hahnemann tells us, in the end, it comes down to vital force.

Not that the concept of "healthy" is a static thing.

Our exact definitions of illness and health are ever changing, both from individual to individual, and also within each individual. Certainly what we considered to be healthy at age twenty is a very different state from what we accept as healthy at age seventy. Our personal definition of health may even change in a matter of days or weeks, most especially under circumstances relating to sudden shock or mechanical trauma.

So both as a human race, and as individuals within that race, our status as "healthy" or "sick" is a part of a continuum. A continuum that shows that the point at which we are healthy and the point at which we are ill is, in no small part, like beauty, in the eye of the beholder. One friend may greet us with words of how well we look, while the next friend warns us to take it easy. And our susceptibility to disease is largely determined by where on that continuum we find ourselves at any given moment.

That person with a strong and unblocked vital force may be said to be at one end of the continuum. This is the person who is simply too strong to easily be made ill. Only the catalysts of the most violent nature or those that are nearly universal in impact will bring him to illness.

On the other end of this continuum is another person who seldom becomes ill, at least not with the ailments that commonly strike others in "average" states of health.

These people may be said to be simply too sick to become ill. Usually they will have a chronic condition that has, over time, so depleted their vital force that the patient is now literally ruled by their condition. And this condition will be so powerfully rooted with that patient's system that it will literally itself block other catalysts from taking root.

Even worse, the patient's vital force may be so very depleted that it no longer reacts to the catalysts of disease as it should. There is nothing left within the patient that will battle for his life against a suspicious intruder.

This often will mean that the weak and chronically ill patient will no longer get colds or other simple acute conditions, or that, even if these acute conditions take hold, that the patient will no longer react to them at all. Far from being the free and healthy person that the individual with strong vital force was, this patient will be held literally in thrall by his chronic complaint and by his weakened vital force.

The vast majority of us are at neither end of the continuum. We are, instead, somewhere in the middle. Our lifestyles are not the best, our diets far from pure. Our systems react to some things, ignore others. In some of us, our system is on hyper-alert, and our defenses arise when they perceive a challenge from what is, in all reality, a benign catalyst. Such is the case for allergies.

In most of us, our internal mechanisms—the vital force and the immune system—are sufficient to ward off most catalysts. The system is sufficiently on appropriate alert and reacts when and how it should. These are the patients whose systems have to either be overwhelmed by a powerful catalyst, in what is most often an acute situation, from mechanical injury or sudden illness, or be slowly broken down over time through a series of smaller illnesses coupled with ongoing stresses in the internal or external environments.

Therefore, most of us are in relatively the same place in terms of our general ability to ward off illness. And it from there becomes a highly individualized matter as to exactly what catalysts and stressors have the ability to call forth the response of disease symptoms from each of us.

Treatment also, at this point, must become a highly individualized matter, and one that reaches the dynamic level of the vital force, the point at which the illness originated and the point at which it can be cured.

That is why so much time and attention must be given to case taking and case management. That is why it is so very important that homeopathic treatments that are undertaken are undertaken carefully and the limits set forth in the Three Laws of Cure.

CHAPTER TWELVE

Goals

Before any sort of homeopathic treatment is undertaken, it is vital that there be an understanding both of the sort of situation that is to be treated and also the goals of that treatment.

There are three distinct forms of homeopathic treatment, each responding to a different sort of situation.

Acute Treatments

The most basic form of treatment speaks to acute situations. In cases requiring acute treatment, the patient experiences a sudden onset of symptoms, to put it simply. But as symptoms are more accurately defined as the patient's responses to changes in his environment, then there is no moment during the patient's life during which he is not experiencing symptoms of one sort or another. During an acute illness, the patient experiences a sudden increase in negative symptoms—those associated with physical, mental, and emotional discomfort.

Acute illnesses tend to come on swiftly and are self-limiting in nature. Which is to say that, in a brief period of time, they tend to resolve themselves. This does not mean that acute illnesses are never serious. The influenza epidemic of the early twentieth century would be categorized as a widespread acute illness, and it killed millions worldwide.

Acute illnesses exist on a continuum from the merely annoying to the violent and deadly. But their very nature has within it a time limitation. Even given the variations in strength and vital force from patient to patient, each will find an end to their illness at about the same period of time.

As Hahnemann himself puts it in aphorism #72 of his *Organon*, "Acute diseases are rapid illness-processes of the abnormally mistuned life principle which are suited to complete their course more or less quickly, but always in a moderate time."

In this definition, Hahnemann reminds us that, as with every other form of dis-

ease, acute illnesses are fundamentally dynamic in nature, involving a blockage or disruption in the vital force.

Treating a patient with an acute illness is a relatively easy thing, most especially
when compared with the skill required to treat the patient who is chronically ill.

When we treat a patient with an acute illness, the goal of that treatment is simple: we seek to restore status quo. In treating a patient with an acute treatment—especially in home treatments for the aches and pains
common to everyday life—an assumption is made
that the patient, before the onset of the illness, was
in a state of relative good health.

> When we treat a patient
> with an acute illness, the
> goal of that treatment
> is simple: we seek to
> restore status quo.

This, of course, may or may not be the actual
case. And in cases in which it is not the reality of
the patient's situation, when the supposed acute
malady is actually just the tip of an iceberg, this assumption can cause problems later
on. Also, in cases in which the apparent acute illness is, in reality, just one in a long
string of supposed acutes that are, when taken into context, a deep chronic condition
that reveals itself periodically, acute treatments can stir up changes in symptoms that
the person administering the treatment may not be equipped to handle.

Even though this assumption of the patient being in good health before the onset
of illness may be far from the truth, it is made every day.

In initiating an acute treatment, the practitioner looks first at the patient as he
existed in that state previous to illness. Then he looks at the patient as he presently
presents himself. And he then isolates the myriad changes that the patient has undergone since the onset of the illness. In giving the homeopathic remedy that is most
similar in its actions to the patient's symptoms, the practitioner attempts to return the
patient to the state he was in before the onset of the illness. No better, no worse. With
the return of status quo, the patient is assumed to be healthy once more and is free to
go about his business.

Because the field of symptoms under consideration is relatively limited—only the
handful of symptoms that have actually changed are considered in the selection of the
remedy—the acute treatment is a relatively simple process. And because the very
nature of the condition, an acute illness, in and of itself limits the length of time during which the patient will be ill, case management is simple as well. One has only to
note the changes made with the first dose of the remedy and then follow the progress
for the period of hours or days during which some sort of continued treatment is
required, whether that be from additional doses of the same remedy, doses of the remedy in a changed potency, or doses of a second or even a third remedy. No matter
what, one has only to conclude the success or failure of the treatment and the lessons
learned in order to close the book on the case.

Along the way, if the illness is found to be truly acute in nature, the practitioner can also count upon the patient's own instincts in treating the case. Hahnemann tells us that the patient who is acutely ill will, with his every instinct, be assisting his body in the restoration of health. His body will have its own strategy of healing. Therefore, the acutely ill patient who craves cold water should be given cold water. The patient whose body is working hard to overcome an acute illness can be trusted in his needs and wants.

It is quite the opposite, as we shall see, for those who are chronically ill.

Constitutional Treatments

About chronic conditions, Hahnemann writes in aphorism #75, "Chronic diseases are those which (each in its own way) dynamically mistune the living organism with small, often unnoticed beginnings. They gradually so remove it from the healthy state . . . that the automatic life energy (called the life force, life principle, or "vital force" [See Chapter 6]), which was ordained to sustain health, opposes them. It does so, both in the beginning and in their continuance, with only imperfect, inexpedient, useless resistance. The life force, which cannot extinguish these diseases by its own power, in and of itself, must allow them to proliferate and it must allow its tuning to be more and more abnormally altered up to the final destruction of the organism."

In the case of chronic illnesses—those that arise slowly, and, without successful treatment, continue a long, slow, and destructive path—therefore, the patient's innate strategy for healing has failed. In these cases, the patient's instincts have been proven to only allow for the continuance of the ailment. The patient's needs and wants should not be granted in these cases, but carefully considered, and, where necessary, denied. In chronic cases, in addition to wise and prudent homeopathic treatment, the patient's dietary cravings and other physical desires may have to be actively countered if he is to be made well.*

The homeopathic treatment used in cases of chronic disease is called *constitutional* treatment, in that it speaks to the whole constitution of the patient. Where acute treatments are given with the implied goal of restoring the patient to the status

---

* Hahnemann actually had very little consideration for those contributed to their own chronic conditions through poor lifestyle choices. In fact, he insisted that these diseases did not actually deserve to be called chronic, since the patient, if he would only pull himself together, could control the progress of the disease. Among his various sore spots were those who "continually expose themselves to *avoidable* malignities," those who "live in unhealthy places," and those who "suffer lack of exercise or open air." He concludes that, "these kinds of ill-health that people bring upon themselves disappear spontaneously under an improved lifestyle, provided no chronic miasm lies in the body. These cannot be called chronic diseases." While I do not think that a kindly physician should say to a patient, "Move out of the damned cellar and then come back for treatment," I do think he has a point.

quo of his former good health, constitutional treatments are undertaken in order to fundamentally improve the quality of the patient's overall health. In these cases, it is not enough that the aches and pains that the patient associates with his condition cease. The patient, after treatment, should not only be free of his disease, but strengthened so that he is less likely to experience that or any other disease in the future.

> Where acute treatments are given with the implied goal of restoring the patient to the status quo of his former good health, constitutional treatments are undertaken in order to fundamentally improve the quality of the patient's overall health.

This is no small goal. And, in the same way, a constitutional treatment is no easy feat. It should, therefore, only be undertaken by those with the skill to see it through to a successful conclusion.

A constitutional treatment may involve the use of several remedies over an extended period of time. It, therefore, requires that the practitioner have the skill to find each remedy and to know when the change from one to another is appropriate. Further, constitutional treatment most often requires a knowledge of potency and dosage as well in the search for the simillimum.

Even the initial case taking itself in a constitutional case is more complex. Where the acute case taking may, in all honestly, consist of a quick look at a scratch or a bump on the head, the constitutional case taking, as will be seen in Chapter 14, involves a good deal of sleuthing in order to ascertain the full range of the patient's symptoms and their metamorphosis over time.

And where the treatment itself in simple acute cases involves only a single arc of action, the treatment required in constitutional care may be as multitiered as the patient's disease. The practitioner may have to follow the patient through a maze of shifts in his symptoms before they are totally cleared.

And remember, one of the clear signs of their clearing once and for all may be a sudden aggravation of symptoms, a period of time in which the patients disease symptoms, which have been resolving themselves for a period of time, will suddenly and inexplicably flare up, causing alarm for both patient and practitioner.

Miasmic Treatment

But there is still a third and deeper level of homeopathic treatment. In order to understand its goals and procedures, you must first understand a new concept—miasms.

The word *miasm* itself means "stain" or "taint." Yasgur's *Dictionary of Homeopathic Medical Terminology* defines miasm simply as "a noxious influence." But the implications of the term extend far beyond these short definitions.

Miasms may be acquired in two ways. First, they may be inherited. In this way, you may think of a miasm in some cases as being a genetic predisposition toward disease, especially of a disease that "runs in the family." Second, a patient may acquire a miasm or miasms during their lifetime. Some are contagious—chiefly through sexually transmitted diseases. Others are the result of violently suppressive allopathic treatment. And still others are the result of one form or other of environmental poisoning. Whatever the cause the result is the same: the patient will display a pronounced predisposition to a specific disease or group of diseases, and the patient may also suffer from a particularly stubborn chronic condition as well. Either way, this is a very difficult patient to cure.

In his lifetime, Hahnemann identified three different miasms. The first was *syphilis*. The second was called *sycosis*, and related to "Figwart disease," or gonorrhea. The third Hahnemann named *psora*.

About psora, in aphorism #80, Hahnemann wrote, "The internal monstrous chronic miasm of psora is immeasurably more widespread, and consequently more significant, than the two chronic miasms just named. While syphilis marks its specific internal wasting sickness with the venereal chancre and sycosis does so with cauliflower-like growth, psora documents itself (only after the complete internal infection of the whole organism) by means of a peculiar skin eruption, sometimes consisting of only a few vesicles, accompanied by an unbearably tickly voluptuous itch and a specific odor. Psora is the true *fundamental* cause and engenderer of almost all the other remaining forms of disease which are numerous, indeed countless."

While it is not the point of this chapter that the reader comes away with a full understanding of the miasms—that would take many more pages than I can dedicate here—I think that it is important to stress that, in his theorizing on the nature of psora, Hahnemann stresses the power of that specific miasm, which he refers to as a "thousand-headed monster." He reports that he dedicated a dozen years of research to understanding the nature of psora and in developing remedies that could combat it.

Since Hahnemann's time, research has continued into the nature of miasms, and in the development of other remedies whose actions could counteract their effects. Each of the miasms can be said to be responsible for myriad afflictions. Each has a set and peculiar path in its destruction. The syphilis miasm, for instance, is known for its wasting diseases, and for the deep, often suicidal, depressions common to those suffering its effects. (Note that I refer to the miasm syphilis here and not to the disease itself. The miasm may be created through suppressive treatment of the disease, or by inheriting the predisposition from one who himself received treatment that made it seem that the disease had been medically cured, when, in reality, only drove it deeper into the body. The doctor giving the suppressive treatment saw the disappearance of the disease as a success, and did not notice the deeper implications of his treatment.)

Of these three miasms, psora is the slowest moving and, in time, the most difficult to untangle. Psora relates to all the mad lifestyle choices we have made, all the many, many suppressive treatments, all the filth in our environment, everything that, bit by bit erodes our ability to live strong and free. It is passed from generation to generation as we, as a species, become ever more tainted through the foolishness of our decisions, the suppressive nature of our medical treatments. With each generation, as the miasm grows stronger, we, as a species, become weaker and more prone to disease. Psora speaks especially of functional diseases, of conditions that no medical test can reveal, and that no sort of treatment can fully resolve. It is the inheritance of the millions of "walking ill," who live their lives narrowed and defined by diseases

> Miasmic treatment seeks to go even deeper than does constitutional treatment. It does not just seek to improve the patient's health—it quite literally seeks to transform the patient into something healthier, something stronger, and something better than he was before.

for which there is no rational cause. Psora is the result of generations opting for the quick fix over the long-term goal. It is the ultimate outcome for the use of that magic leaf.

Miasmic treatment seeks to go even deeper than does constitutional treatment. It does not just seek to improve the patient's health—it quite literally seeks to transform the patient into something healthier, something stronger and something better than he was before.

This is a form of treatment best left to the most dedicated and highly skilled practitioners. Only they will have the ability to see it through to a successful conclusion.

Inverse Proportions

At this point, now that I have identified all three levels of homeopathic treatment and the goals associated with each, I want to note that, in my experience, the number of remedies used, as well as the number of specific doses tends to be in sort of an inverse proportion with the depth of the patient's condition. In other words, the patient with an acute disease may require more different remedies and more doses of each than will the patient with a chronic condition, or the patient requiring miasmic treatment.

The deeper the illness, the more likely that the doses of remedies given will be further and further apart. The more deeply the symptoms of illness have grafted themselves onto the patient, the more gingerly they must be removed. Where a serious acute condition may require quick and decisive action, a deep chronic condition needs gentle nudging and time in which to rewrite the cycles of pain.

Therefore, the practitioner who is chiefly skilled in acute treatments* may make use of many more remedies over a shorter period of time than the practitioner treating constitutionally will in a period of months or years. (In fact, one may say that this is one of the dangers present in shortsightedly treating a chronic condition as a series of separate acute illnesses. In that the acute treatment allows for a bit more latitude in treatment, the patient may end up over medicated from the many remedies he has received. It should be remembered that, even in acute cases, the Law of Minimum is still intact.)

Understanding the Goal of Treatment

Before any homeopathic treatment of any sort is entered into, I think that it is important that the patient and practitioner alike agree on the specific goals of that treatment. A patient may, for instance, suffer from a chronic respiratory condition that presents itself annually as a series of colds. And they may come for help with this specific cold. I believe that, in this case, before the practitioner begins a constitutional cure, he must fully explain the situation as he sees it to the patient and make sure that the patient gives fully informed permission before proceeding. If that patient is comfortable only with a simple acute treatment, if he only wants help with this cold and is not ready yet to tackle anything deeper, then the practitioner must decide if he can abide by that decision. If he can, then his job has become easier. If not, he can send the patient off to another practitioner's office.

In the same way, it is never proper for the practitioner to take it upon himself to reach down and treat a miasm that he suspects is the root cause of the patient's illness

---

* And I do believe that there is such a thing as a practitioner who is more skilled, who thinks more clearly when dealing out acute treatments. In the same way, I also believe that others are more gifted in working with constitutional care. In fact, quite honestly, I have never known a single practitioner who I considered to be equally skilled with both acute and constitutional care. And, while I'm on the subject, let me just note that I feel that homeopathic organizations and medical professionals who relegate the practice of acute care to lay people, while solely granting medical professionals the right to work constitutionally are making an arbitrary and somewhat nearsighted separation of tasks. I have known some laypeople with a skill for constitutional treatment that would leave the professionals in the dust. In the same vein, let me note that I in no way consider acute care to be a lesser thing than is constitutional. While the goal may be simpler, the circumstances are often far more dramatic than the case taking professionals ever see in their offices. The acute practitioner—layperson or medical professional—has to think quickly and clearly and act decisively and correctly. Not an easy thing. Where those taking the constitutional case may get out their texts and computers, the practitioner dealing with a screaming baby had better have the knowledge needed right inside their brain. Allopathic medicine does not make this mistake. It recognizes that the doctors in the ER are practicing a different sort of medicine that requires a different sort of practitioner. Homeopaths, take note.

without first explaining the situation as he sees it to the patient and receiving an agreement to proceed.

Only when the patient and the practitioner can work together as a team in a relationship based on mutual respect and honesty, and only when they can be sure that they are each working toward the same goal, can the patient be hopeful of a successful outcome.

We, therefore, have to next learn how we can establish a healing team, with a common purpose and goal, in order to get the job done.

CHAPTER THIRTEEN

Teamwork

Any situation, any interaction between two people, contains four types of information. There is the information that I know but you don't. There is the information that you know but I don't. There is the information that both of us know. And
there is the information that neither of us knows.

To apply this concept to medical treatment of any sort, especially homeopathic
treatment, is to understand that the medical process is most effective when it is a
team effort.

In that there is a good deal about every illness that neither the patient nor the
practitioner will ever know—for instance, exactly the source of the illness or its
meaning on the deepest levels of being—it is important that the practitioner, his
patient, and all others concerned about and impacted by the illness work hard
together in order to bring about a cure.

It is important that they form a healing team.

The Healing Team

In any situation involving more than one person, things function much more
smoothly if each person involved understands and accepts his function within the
group. In homeopathic case taking, things work best if three roles are filled, although
as few as two or as many as you wish may fill them. Two of these roles are objective in
nature, which is to say, they stand outside the "action" and witness it. Both record the
information given as best they can without interpretation. One of these two is dispassionate, the other compassionate. The third role is completely subjective. It lives outside the realm of fact, and is asked, instead, to simply tell the truth as he knows it. The
person filling this role is, after all, the patient.

The Patient

The role of the patient is rather similar to that of the honored guest at a banquet, if only in that all eyes are focused on him, all attention is his.

In any form of medicine, the patient is the only source of subjective information concerning the illness. Only the patient can give a true notion as to how the illness has impacted his system, from onset to the point of treatment. Only he can reveal the intangibles of the case, how the symptoms have changed him emotionally and mentally, what makes his symptoms feel better or worse, how his symptoms have changed or moved since the onset of the illness, what he was doing, feeling, or thinking prior to the onset of his illness. The problem is that, in medical models other than the homeopathic, this wealth of information is virtually ignored in favor of technological tools and medical tests. The fact that the patient experienced his sore throat first on the left side of this throat, before it moved to the right is of no interest for the allopath. Meanwhile, the homeopath may find that bit of information, when considered along side of all the other bits of information that have been gathered, sufficient enough to select the remedy Lachesis over other remedies associated with patients with sore throats, like Lycopodium or Phosphorus.

In the process of case taking, the patient needs to give the practitioner what information he can concerning the case. It is helpful, of course, if the patient can speak rationally and can give clear information. But I hesitate to ever ask a patient to make an attempt to do so, to be anything other than he is naturally in the given situation, because the patient's behavior under the stress of illness can be very telling.

Therefore, it is the patient's role in case taking simply to present himself as he is. And to let be known all that he is feeling and thinking. If, for instance, he does not want to be touched if the practitioner wishes to examine him, he should let that be known clearly. Simply put, at the time of case taking, it is most important that the patient simply be himself and react to his circumstances with complete honesty. The practitioner who attempts to fit the patient into a particular mold, who wants to control the nature in which the patient presents himself is changing the nature of the case taking, and may, in doing so, rig the results.

After the case taking, the patient is perhaps even more important to the curative process. His role now changes from a rather passive one in which he simply presents the truth of his condition, to an active role in which he becomes a full partner with his practitioner. Where patients under allopathic care are required only to let their doctors know if the side effects experienced while taking medication are too difficult to bear, or if something traumatic has happened, like blood in their stool, the patient working with a homeopath will be expected to report the full range of changes that they experience while under care: good, bad, or indifferent. Every nuance may contain informative facts. The patient's subjective information may be key in guiding the practitioner in continued treatment. For this reason, it is very important that the relationship between the patient and the practitioner be one that allows for honesty, one that is based on mutual trust.

After having been involved solely with homeopathy for a period of more than twenty years, I recently had reason to consult an allopathic physician. After the initial visit, I returned for my follow-up, and, in true homeopathic fashion, began telling the doctor about all that I had experienced as a result of my treatment. After a few seconds, I realized that my information was not only not needed in that doctor's opinion, but that it was unwanted as well. The doctor took my report personally, in that my experience had been, for the most part, highly negative. He interrupted me and spent the rest of the visit explaining to me that his treatment was my only option, implying that, therefore, I had to pretty much decide to like it.

> More than anything else . . . the patient should simply experience his ailment and share, as best he can, all that he experiences with his practitioner.

I never went back.

Allopathic medicine is a very different thing from homeopathy.

More than anything else, the patient who is being treated homeopathically must be truthful. Not only should he report his situation as he is experiencing it, but he should also embody the truth of that situation. The patient should simply experience his ailment and share, as best he can, all that he experiences with his practitioner.

The Physician

In homeopathic medicine, the practitioner takes on the role of the physician, with all its implied responsibilities. This is the role of the dispassionate observer. By this I do not mean that the physician doesn't care whether or not the patient achieves his cure. This could not be further from the truth. What I mean is that, when in the role of the dispassionate observer, the physician refuses to enter into the drama of the situation.

The physician must be clear minded and clear sighted. He must observe all that is going on around him. He must be prepared to take in and record all the information that the patient is revealing about himself and his illness, while at the same time stay present with the patient as he speaks. The physician who buries his head in note taking, or who concerns himself with checking reference books during the case taking is, in disconnecting his full attention from his patient, weakening his ability to select the needed remedy.

Some homeopaths have, in recent years, made use of technology to video tape their case takings, so that the exact words of the patient can be recalled, as can their behavior and mannerisms. This frees the physician to give full attention to the case at hand and not to note taking.

The role of the physician after and beyond the case taking remains much the same. The physician is not in any way to be elevated above the patient—is never to take on that paternalistic role so common in allopathic medicine. Instead the physician and patient should act as partners in seeking a cure for the patient's ails. Each should contribute to this common goal with equal care and honesty.

I often think that patients are, when they visit an allopath, renting a doctor. They are exchanging money for their doctor's time and expertise. It does not in any way matter what the doctor thinks of the patient and the patient of the doctor. Indeed, in many of today's medical practices, the patient may rarely, if ever, see the same doctor twice. No, in allopathic medicine, technology is king. Since the function of the doctor is largely to decide what medical tests need taking and, based upon their results and the ultimate diagnosis, to choose which of the medicines usually associated with the diagnosed condition the patient should take, the relationship between the doctor and patient is perfunctory at best.*

Again, homeopathic medicine is different.

Because of this, I make it a practice never to recommend a homeopath to a potential patient. Instead, I try to teach what a patient should rightfully be able to expect from a homeopath and then trust that the patient, with some effort, will find the best possible practitioner for his own needs and wants.

I never make recommendations because there is something necessary in the interplay between homeopath and patient that cannot be predicted. A particular well-trained and highly skilled homeopath may simply be the wrong practitioner for a given patient. Because of this, I believe that trying to put together a patient and a homeopath is sort of like arranging a blind date. Two really great people may find that they just don't like each other. And since, in my experience, the relationship between the homeopath and the patient requires a level of respect, trust, and intimacy that does not exist in the allopathic medical model, I tend to stay away from these recommendations, since, like those blind dates, they tend to blow up in your face.

Of course, we pay our homeopaths just as we do our allopaths. But, even with the exchange of money, the dynamic is different. When you enter into a homeopath's practice, you are setting up a relationship with that individual homeopath, and not with his office. I would not more be willing to go to see my homeopathic practitioner, only to find that I have been handed off to someone else in his office, than I would be willing to see my child handed over to just any teacher or nanny. Homeopaths belong

---

* I have noticed, for instance, that whenever I find myself in an allopath's office, I am asked by the doctor where I went to college. It occurred to me recently that, in the many years since I graduated from college, it is only in allopathic medical offices that I am asked where I went. Is this because he went to Yale and I didn't? Or is it because he has been taught in medical school that this is a safe topic for conversation during the exam?

to that category of professionals in our lives with whom we build real bonds, despite the fact that one is in one way or another paying the other for his services. And, as with the teacher/student bond, in the bond between a homeopath and a patient there can be mutual healing and growth.

To be effective in his practice, a homeopath must be capable of having true concern for the well-being of his patients without ever letting a patient, in a true state of fear or anger, dictate the terms of the treatment. They must never allow their patient's fears to affect them, only observe the fact that the patient has them. They must remain outside that emotional setting, observing it, learning from it. Remember, in homeopathic medicine,

> . . . the relationship between the homeopath and the patient requires a level of respect, trust, and intimacy that does not exist in the allopathic medical model.

the practitioner's role is not to treat the disease, but, instead, to treat the patient with the disease. Therefore, the exact manner in which the patient reacts to that disease—in terms of the sum total of his physical symptoms, his emotional state and his mental/verbal skills—will guide the practitioner to the remedy that can set things straight.

The Caregiver

The role of the caregiver balances that of the practitioner. Where the practitioner is objective in viewpoint and remains dispassionate throughout, the caregiver is both objective and compassionate.

The caretaker, therefore, fulfills two functions. First, they act as the patient's advocate, supporting the patient throughout the case taking and treatment. Second, they act as another source of information for the practitioner, one that may even be more valuable than is the patient himself. In that the person taking on the role of caregiver is most often a parent, sibling, or mate to the patient, the caregiver is in the unique position of knowing the patient well—knowing their usual patterns of behavior and lifestyle when the patient is not sick, and, often just how those patterns have shifted as the patient moved into illness—and yet they stand apart from the patient. This gives the caregiver unique insights into the case, insights that neither the practitioner nor the patient himself can know.

For both these reasons, it may be important for the caregiver to be present both during the initial case taking and during follow-up visits. If the patient is too young or too ill to be given instructions concerning his care, the caregiver, as his advocate, must be given this information. The caregiver may also be the person entrusted with the administration of homeopathic remedies throughout treatment, just as they may also be the person who sees to it that the patient has nourishing foods on hand and that he eats them.

Finally, through careful observation of the interplay between the patient and the caregiver, the practitioner may be given insights into the patient's lifestyle and how it possibly impacts the case. All things considered, the caregiver's role is just as important to the curative process as is the practitioner or the patient. It is just as important, therefore, that the caregiver understands his role and be willing to see it through until the end of treatment.

Mixed Roles

Homeopathic treatment can become a good deal more complicated when situations dictate that the three roles that make up the healing team be filled by only two people.

If, for instance, as is commonly the case in home treatment, the practitioner is also the patient's caregiver, then the single person fulfilling this dual role is going to have to be capable of being dispassionate when necessary and very compassionate when that response is needed. This can be very taxing for the parent who is himself or herself in a state of shock over a beloved child's sudden serious illness. It can be very difficult indeed for this parent to "step aside" from his or her emotions and think clearly enough to diagnose the case and select the appropriate remedy. Certainly, at the same time it should be noted that the patient who has a practitioner who is also their caregiver is a patient with a practitioner who is most dedicated to their cure, and who will stop at nothing to see that the cure takes place. The patient who has a practitioner/caregiver who can assume each role as needed is a very lucky patient indeed.

Further difficulties arise when the patient finds himself in circumstances in which he must function as his own caregiver. In this case, the practitioner receives no outside information in the case taking, only the subjective information that the patient has to offer. And, further, the patient who is in charge of his own dosing is likely to take more doses than necessary. An objective caregiver can more easily know when the time has come for the second dose than can the patient himself, as the patient's own decision-making ability likely is warped by fear and pain.

And yet both of these possibilities arise very often. Often illness strikes late in the night or under other circumstances that require immediate action. In these cases, the needed action must be taken by the caregiver by acting as practitioner as well.

In the same way, millions of people in this country live alone and must take care of themselves when they are sick. If they don't make their own chicken soup no one else is going to. In these cases, the practitioner must make very certain that he instructs the patient well in his own care and in the appropriate taking of his remedy. If not, a spoiled treatment can easily result.

In some rare instances, the patient may have to be his own homeopath as well as his own caregiver. It goes without saying that this is a circumstance to be avoided if at all possible. The dynamic between practitioner and patient is so vital to cure that it should be sought whenever possible. But, if circumstances dictate that the patient must find his own remedy, then he must do so with as clear a mind as possible and must avoid the temptation to just try remedy after remedy, as he, with a mind clouded by his illness, attempts to find the right remedy. In fact, if the condition is something beyond the simplest bump on the head, I would find it far preferable for the patient to seek allopathic aid than to try to be his own homeopath.

Maintaining the Roles

No matter the case or the number of people involved, it is absolutely necessary that each person understand the role that they are to fulfill and agree to take it on to the best of their ability from the onset of treatment until that treatment is concluded. Anyone who has acted in the role of the practitioner or the caregiver—to say nothing of the patient—can tell you just how difficult it can be to fulfill a role that may require more time, emotion, and energy than you feel that it is yours to give. However, I feel that great harm can come to the patient who feels himself abandoned either by his practitioner or his caregiver.

Therefore, the members of the team have to be in place to stay. And they have to always keep their eyes on the goal of cure and that, in doing so, each fulfills their role to the best of their ability. This means that worries over money or old emotional baggage between the patient and the caregiver must be put aside for a time, if not forgiven once and for all. That is, in fact, how a healing of relationships may take place during the time of cure. And that is how the smoothest and the deepest homeopathic cure is going to take place.

CHAPTER FOURTEEN

Case Taking

The opening line of one of Joan Didion's best novels, *A Book of Common Prayer*, is a simple sentence. "I will be her witness." Joan Didion would have made a hell of a homeopath.

In his book *Language in Thought and Action*, S. I. Hayakawa informs us that we "cannot *not* communicate."*

When you take a homeopathic case, keep both of these statements in mind. Remember that your purpose is to be the patient's witness. And that the process of case taking is an act of communication—a process that is always happening, but not always verbal.

The case taker's primary job is to witness the patient in his or her wholeness. This takes more than a willingness to listen to the patient and dutifully record what he or she says. Although that can certainly be part of the job.

No, the job of the case taker is to record the whole of the patient's being, if you will. This first requires that you enter into the process without judgment, either of the patient or of what the patient may need in terms of a remedy. (In order to avoid early judgments, I tend never to look at any intake form that might tell me the nature of the patient's complaints or anything about them. Just watch how they walk in the room, how they sit, what they are wearing. Notice if they have any particular scent, from perfume to body odor. Notice anything unusual about them, from their make-up

---

* If you have never read Hayakawa's book, I would strongly suggest that you do so before you ever do any homeopathic case taking. The book was born in 1938 as a course outline for a Freshman English class at the University of Wisconsin. The original title was "Language in Thought." The title evolved as the book, in *Organon* fashion, itself grew from a set of mimeographed pages to one of the classic texts on semantics. It was first published in 1939 by Harcourt Brace & Company. In that you can never be too rich, too thin, or communicate too effectively, I would suggest that you put a copy of this book among your homeopathic reference books. After all, the importance of effective communication in case taking cannot be overstated.

to their facial expression.) From the moment that the patient walks in the door until they have closed it behind them, it is the role of the case taker to record all data possible, not just the list of the patient's ailments.

So, if you are the sort of person who is easily distracted, or who tends to look out the window, or at your fingernails, or, worst of all, over a person's left shoulder, while you are speaking with someone, then perhaps homeopathy is not for you. At least from the case-taking standpoint.

Models for Taking a Case

In the allopathic medical model, the give and take between the doctor and patient is paternalistic in nature. The doctor is given the father's role. He sits behind his big desk while the patient has a small chair opposite. When he physically examines the patient, the doctor remains armored in his full business attire, while the patient is reduced to disrobing or wearing a thin paper gown. The interchange between the two is set in stone, with the doctor asking questions and the patient answering them. The full visit usually breaks down into three parts: a brief greeting, during which the patient is asked the nature of his complaint; an examination, during which the doctor explores the patient's body for some verification of the complaint; and the final interview, during which the doctor tells the patient of his findings or lack of same, and then, more often than not, the patient is sent off to a clinic where blood can be taken and specific medical tests performed. On the basis of those test results, the doctor reveals his plan of action to the patient, either by phone or in a second visit. From there prescriptions are called in and insurance companies billed.

Under the homeopathic model, things are quite different.

As outlined in the last chapter, the relationship between homeopath and patient is more of a partnership. In many ways they speak as peers, in that the homeopath understands and respects that the knowledge the patient has concerning his own body and how it works, to say nothing of the specifics of the case at hand, is far greater than anything that the homeopath could ever gather on his own, with or without medical testing.

A proper homeopathic prescription could not more be made solely on the basis of a blood test than it could on the basis of the disease diagnosis alone. Neither of these can give the facts that individualize the case—the exact symptoms, the onset and the nature of each. Without a thorough knowledge of the patient and his own peculiar experience of his disease, homeopathic treatments could be no more specific, and, therefore, no more effective than are allopathic medicine.

Gathering information concerning the patient and his symptoms is what case taking is all about. There is, therefore, no way to overstate the importance of this process. As homeopath James Tyler Kent put it, "A case well taken is half cured."

Taking the Case

Case taking is the gathering of information directly related to the disease symptoms that the patient is experiencing. In some simple acute situations, that may well be enough. But in deeper cases, cases involving more complex acutes and all chronic complaints, the practitioner will need more information, information concerning the patient's lifestyle (with thorough information on the environments in which he lives and works), his medical history (most especially including information on what allopathic treatments he has undergone and their results), and the patterns by which he lives his life in times of good health and how those patterns have shifted with the onset of illness.

In gathering these symptoms, it is important that the practitioner gain a complete knowledge of both the subjective and the objective symptoms pertaining to the case.

The objective symptoms are those that will, in some way, be apparent to the practitioner, even if the patient himself is unaware of them. A particular discoloration of the skin, for instance, may be an example of a telling objective symptom. And examination of the affected part or parts of the body may well yield a great amount of objective information. And, again in the case of a simple acute situation like a mechanical injury, this may be all the information that you need in order to select the appropriate remedy. A verbal exchange—that which is often called "the Interview" in homeopathic jargon—may be limited to just a few basic questions ("How did it happen?" "Does this hurt?" "If so, how?" "What is the quality of the pain?" etc.) or may not be needed at all.*

To put it simply: please let the case taking suit the case. Some homeopaths approach their cases like Nancy Drew did her mysteries, all giggly at the prospect of

---

* I have to express a personal opinion here that, most especially in the United States, modern homeopaths tend to take the case for so long and in such depth that, ultimately, they cannot make use of all the information gleaned in the process of choosing an effective remedy. In my opinion, enough information should be gathered so that the practitioner can be confident in his or her choice of a remedy. No more and no less. Certainly, having a solid amount of information is necessary, but, in truth, it sometimes seems that practitioners have turned case taking into a vaudeville. More and more it seems to involve pulling a long string of multicolored silk handkerchiefs from the practitioner's sleeve, or pulling a magical rabbit out of a hat, instead of a process of rather simple communication that results in a successful treatment. By the time we have asked the patient what his grandfather preferred for breakfast, eggs or oatmeal, we have simply gone too far. The same may be said of the intake forms that some practitioners have their patients fill out before they even see them. Case taking is really a very simple thing. I think that if we could get homeopaths to turn off their computers and close their books during the case taking and actually pay attention to their patients that we might be well on the way to a better practice of medicine.

unraveling the case. Sometimes Junior has fallen down and bumped his head. It is just not necessary to know what his grandfather died from in order to treat him.

Case taking is a verbal as well as a non-verbal process. It begins when the patient and practitioner first meet. It continues until one leaves the room or until it is declared finished. It is a process by which the practitioner can try and determine on a physical level the progress of the disease and its impact on his body. On an emotional and mental level, the process is the same. The practitioner is seeking information as to the changes that have occurred along with the disease.

> Case taking is a verbal as well as a non-verbal process. It begins when the patient and practitioner first meet. It continues until one leaves the room or until it is declared finished.

As I have said in my classes over the years, in choosing the correct remedy, it is less important that we know the model of the bus that hit the patient. It is more important that we know what the patient did when he was hit by a bus. Did he cry? Did he scream in agony? Did he blame the bus or blame himself? Did he shake his fist in the air and swear revenge? In other words, it is often more important, in structuring treatment, to know how the patient has reacted within the circumstances of his illness than it is to know all about the illness itself.

For complex cases, this involves a blend of subjective and objective information. It means that we have to gather the information that the patient has locked within himself, as well as the information that he is wearing on his sleeve, or, in the case of a black eye, on his face.

That's what a case taking is and what it attempts to do. I don't know if it is possible to give any more specific information about case taking. I don't even think that it is possible to give an exact lesson plan in good case taking. It is more something that is learned, again through trial and error, through clinical experience in dealing with real patients in real situations. In time, each homeopath finds the method of case taking that works best for him. In time, each learns to judge the amount of information required in order for them to take the case to conclusion.

What I can do in these pages is to give some guidelines that can be considered when a case is taken. Here are a few of the most important:

- First, the practitioner should not talk too much. The case taking, whether the situation is acute or chronic should start with a very simple question. "What happened?" works well enough in the case of simple mechanical injuries. But even the most complex case should begin with as simple a question as "How may I help you?"

- The practitioner should never ask leading questions. I believe that about the worst thing you can do is assume *anything* in a case taking. This means that the homeopath who, based on the patient's clothing or demeanor or hairstyle or perfume, makes assumptions about what remedy they might need is treading on some very thin ice. While this sort of detail may be very valuable in confirming a remedy choice, it should not, on its own, be the chief reason for a remedy's selection. Even the most well-meaning homeopath may just get it into their head too early on in a case taking that the patient needs a specific remedy. If the assumption of a needed remedy triggers leading questions about which the practitioner has already made assumptions concerning the answers, then the whole process of case taking has been tainted.

- Case taking is never the time during which the practitioner should be trying to show the patient how smart he is or how modern his tools are. Play with your computer later. Put away your need to let the patient know that you know ever so much more about homeopathy than he does by interrupting or correcting. You will show them how great you are when you give them the correct remedy.

- In the same way, a case taking is not a time during which it is appropriate for the practitioner to let the patient know just how charming or witty he is. The patient is the one on whom we are all supposed to be focusing. Anything, including a sparkling sense of humor, that detracts from the patient and places the attention on the practitioner is simply out of place.

- Allow silences to happen. Many homeopaths, maybe with the hope of getting on with the next case, go right to their next question the moment that the patient slows down for a moment. I have found that more information comes out of an awkward silence, when the practitioner is just sitting there looking at the patient, and saying nothing for a long moment than from anything else. In that moment of quiet, the patient will often say something of great value—quite often something that they have been reluctant to say or admit. Remember, the case taker's role is to guide, to observe, and record and, above all else, to listen.*

- Always make sure that the patient has said his piece. In fact, at the beginning of the case taking, when the patient is telling you how you can help them, never

---

* I believe that, very often, the patient's journey back to health begins, not with the taking of a remedy, but within the process of case taking. When the patient is listened to, when his history, his thoughts and his worries (to say nothing of his symptoms) are truly heard and taken seriously, you can quite often see not only the beginning of hope of that patient's face but also the beginning of the healing process itself. It is essential that homeopaths learn to truly and actively listen to their patients. This is especially true in case involving chronic conditions and constitutional or miasmic care.

interrupt. Never ask for clarification at this point. If there is something that you will have to return to later, note it. Pay attention to what the patient is saying. When they finish telling you their symptoms, I always find it useful to ask, "Anything else?" There may be a good deal more that the patient, in the interest of time or out of discomfort or intimidation, is not addressing.

• Speaking of discomfort or intimidation, the practitioner that does not, before the case taking even begins, create an environment in which the patient can be both physically and emotionally comfortable is one hell of a lousy practitioner. Like a good hostess will create an environment of joy for her guests, the practitioner must create an environment of safety, acceptance, and comfort for his patients. And just as the patient will, from the moment they enter the room, be communicating their case with the practitioner, if only they will stop and pay attention, in the same way, from the very first moment the practitioner is communicating a good deal about himself with his patient. He communicates his opinion of himself, his opinion of his patient, and the degree to which he is dedicated to the healing process.

Okay, you are the practitioner and you have just met the patient and he has answered your initial questions by telling you why he is in your office and what he wants from you. By telling you in some detail what is wrong with him that he needs help. You have listened carefully and recorded what you must of the information given, either by taking discrete notes (the patient should never feel as if they are being interviewed for the local paper by a newsman with a spiral notebook), or by recording the session (with full consent from the patient, of course).

You allowed for the awkward silence at the end of the monologue portion of the patient's case, and were careful not to interrupt him. Now you are going to have to go back and get the details that were left out in the monologue.

You are going to have to know the same sort of information about each of the individual symptoms that the patient mentioned. The information needed will include:

• The onset of the symptom: What the patient was doing or thinking or otherwise experiencing at the time the symptom came on? What foods might they have been eating before the onset of the symptom? If this is a symptom that reoccurs, try to get at the pattern of what might trigger that symptom.

• The location of the symptom: It is important to know more than just that the patient has a headache. Where, specifically in the head does it occur? If the headache reoccurs, does it always take place in the same part of the head—the right side, or the top, or the forehead, or whatever? Or does the headache locate itself differently each time? Does the headache move? Does it start on the right side of the forehead and move left? And how does the moving or changing of the location of the pain affect the pain? Does it grow worse as it moves, or better or stay the same?*

- The sensation of the symptom: If it causes pain, what type of pain does it cause?

- How long has the pain lasted? If this is a reoccurring symptom, ask how long it usually lasts. Seek the pattern of the symptom in terms of duration.

- What makes that symptom feel better? What makes it feel worse? While the symptom is present, does the patient have any cravings or desires? Does he want to drink cold water when he has his headache? Is there anything that he cannot bear while the symptom is present? Does he find that he cannot bear the sight or smell of food when his head hurts?

- What has the patient already tried in terms of other treatments, allopathic or homeopathic, for this symptom? What was the outcome of each of those treatments?

After you have looked at each of the patient's symptoms, then it is time to try and figure out how the symptoms—assuming that the case is complex enough that the patient suffers from more than one—interact with each other.

It can be very helpful to also know the order in which the symptoms appeared. Which came first, then second, and so on.

In the same way, it is important to try and understand how the symptoms relate to each other. Do two symptoms always occur together, or does one particular symptom always appear just before the other one starts? Does one particular symptom always mean that another one is about to start?

If the patient has not as yet shared with you the emotional ramifications of this ailment, and if they are not apparent by his behavior, it may also be very important to ask, "How does this all make you feel?"

The practitioner will want some general knowledge of the patient as well. He will want to know the patient's lifestyle, his diet, and the amount of exercise he takes in a given period of time. Most important will be the patient's likes and dislikes. What does he crave in terms of diet, or in relationships? What pleases him?

In the same way, the practitioner will want to know what displeases the patient. What things, people, or situations does he really hate? Strong likes and dislikes can be guides that lead you to the right remedy selection.

---

* Lots of questions about a headache, I know. But this is the information that will help you in the selection of the remedy. It is important, however, that you don't ask these questions as I have written them here. Again, we don't want to lead the patient with a barrage of questions. Instead, ask, "Where in the head does the headache occur?" and take if from there.

When you feel that you have exhausted the interview process, or when you think that you have gathered sufficient information to guide you to a remedy, there is still one more question that you have to ask. It is very important. Ask the patient, "Is there anything that I haven't mentioned that you want to tell me?" You may be surprised what answers come from that question. At the very least, the patient will tell you that they are satisfied that they have had the chance to fully and completely tell you everything that they think is important for you to know (and, likely, a good more besides), and that they feel that they have been listened to and heard. I strongly believe that it is very important that every patient feels that they have been heard and that what they have said has been honored and truly listened to. Again, this is, to me, an important part of the healing process and one that all too often is lacking in the field of medicine.

Case Taking with All Your Senses

Up until now, I have only mentioned the actual interview part of case taking, and have all but ignored the examination of the patient.

More often than not, especially in household care, the examination involves nothing more than looking at the particular scratch or bump that is, in and of itself, the reason for treatment.

But in any case taking, it may be important for the practitioner to examine the part of the body affected by the symptom. The exact nature of the examination should, of course, be determined both by the location of the injury and by the level of professional skill possessed by the practitioner. In the case of a medical professional, a thorough clinical examination may be called for. Some modern homeopaths may also wish to make use of technological tools or medical tests as well—although the information yielded by such testing will be used in a different manner than an allopath would use it.

The most important point here is that the practitioner, in examining his patient, must make use of all his senses—or nearly all, as we shall see.

The practitioner must use his eyes from the first moment that he meets the patient. He may need them to visually examine a particular part of the patient's body as well.

The practitioner must make good use of his ears, hearing not only the patient's words, but also his other utterances, his sighs, his laughter, and so forth. In the same way, he should listen not only to what the patient is saying, but also how he is saying it. He must listen to the emotional content of the patient's words.

The practitioner must use his sense of touch. When he greets the patient, the strength or weakness of the patient's handshake may be very telling. And, if the patient is to be physically examined, the practitioner may need to touch the patient repeatedly in order to palpate specific areas of the patient's body.

Then there is the sense of smell. Often cases can be solved by smell alone. The practitioner who knows the peculiar smell given off by a Thuja patient will recognize it when he smells it. In the same way, by smell alone a Mercurius case may be solved. Even in a more general way, the sense of smell can help the practitioner to gather information. The pronounced smell of mothballs or perfume may help the practitioner to know the cause of the patient's symptoms.

I know that I said that the practitioner must make use of all his senses. But, in truth, I have never found an appropriate use for the sense of taste in the case taking process. In that no good can come from tasting your patient, I suggest you leave it out.

Ordering the Symptoms

I know that other texts may tell you that it is very important that you order the symptoms in some specific manner. Some will tell you that, based on Hering's Law, you should list the symptoms from the top of the patient's head downward. Others will tell you to order them from the most recent backward to the earliest symptom.

I don't think much of the first method, in that I think it is an artificial organization and one that will not help you later in trying to take this information and make sense of it. While Hering's Law is a valuable guideline with which we can observe how healing takes place, it is not of value in case taking. While Hering has outlined for us the general direction in which a healing will take place, the human patient seems never to fit neatly into any specific format while healing. (For a description of Hering's Law, see Chapter 10.) Instead, we need to keep our attention firmly fixed on the patient and his or her own specific experience of illness and health.

Personally, I find that what works best is to trust the patient and go with the order of symptoms that he gives you in the interview. While it is certainly true that the particular symptom or symptoms that forced him to seek help may be the least of his problems, and the least important in actually ultimately finding a remedy, it should be remembered that this symptom was the one that the patient found troubling enough to try and rid himself of with your help. Therefore, I always start with that symptom. In doing so, I feel that I am respecting the patient and trusting him in what he finds important.

From there, I tend to go as the interview goes. I follow the maze of the symptoms as they are presented to me. If, however, the patient suddenly remembers something and interjects—excitedly or passionately—some information concerning a new symptom, I may mark it as being of especial interest. Again, let the case taking suit the needs of the patient and the situation in which he finds himself, and not your own needs and wants.

At the end of the case taking, after you and the patient have parted, take some time and consider what you have witnessed. Then make some notes. What stood out to you? What did you particularly notice about this person? Was it the way he walked, or spoke, or was it the way in which he talked about a particular symptom? Again, strong emotions—pro or con—can be very important. And things that have the power to change other symptoms or things for the better or for the worse should be noted. They can be very important as well.

I personally try to take as few notes as possible during the interview, while still recording what I must. I especially find it useful to try and record as much information as possible in the patient's own words. These words, if well recorded, can lead to some very important discoveries about the patient's case. In fact, there is a homeopathic text entitled *Sensations As If,* which was written back in 1937 by Dr. Herbert A. Roberts. It lists the most idiosyncratic phrases, all of which you may well hear coming out of the patient's mouth. The patient may, for instance, say that they feel as if they had a "bee humming in my head." A quick look at the text would tell you that you better consider the remedy Sulphur, because the patients needing that remedy say just that phrase.

Not only do you want to capture the patient's exact words and phrasing while you are taking his case, you want to capture some idea of exactly who he is as a person. What motivates him? What emotions come easily to him, and what emotions are more difficult? How well is he coping with his illness? How much does it limit his life? How has he changed as a person since the onset of the illness, as opposed to how he has changed in specific characteristics or aspects of his life because of his pain?

I know that it will not be possible to come to such a deep understanding of every patient. And, as I have said before, I know that in many cases it will not be necessary to understand much of anything other than that the bee stung the patient and the sting is itchy and red and swelling.

But, when needed, I think that this is where the emphasis should be, in understanding the patient as a being first and then in understanding how he has changed, both in the details of his symptoms and then as a whole being, through his experience with his disease. The practitioner who tries to reduce his patient to a series of symptoms is denying the full nature of his patient and shortchanging his patient in terms of care.

Third Parties and Case Taking

If the patient's caregiver is part of this case taking, then it is important that the practitioner makes the best use of their presence without letting them in any way interfere with the process.

It is important, for instance, that the practitioner remains in charge of the case taking at all times, and that the caregiver, in their rather passionate role of patient advocate, never be allowed to seize the reins.

Nor should they ever be allowed to interrupt the patient. What the caregiver has to say may be very important, but, if they cannot add to the discussion appropriately, it may be necessary for the practitioner to suggest that he have a brief conversation with the patient alone and that he will then have one with the caregiver. Caregivers who are also parents can be extremely helpful to the case taking. They can fill in information that the young patient simply cannot provide. But in the same way they can be troublemakers as well, especially when they are allowed to correct the patient, or to interrupt their flow of language in order to interject information of their own.

Learning to deal with the three-party case taking can take some time and effort. But, when it has been mastered and the practitioner can both listen to two other people and keep track of what they have said, and, at the same time, stay in control of the circumstances that surround the case taking, then the information yielded can be well worth the extra work required.

Case Taking and Cure

I've already quoted Kent in saying that "A case well taken is half cured," or words to that effect. But I want to drive that point home once more.

You may only have, with any given patient, one chance to get the gist of the case and then find the remedy to solve it. Circumstances may dictate that treatment must come now or never. Or you may be faced with a patient who, for whatever reason, is simply not going to be willing to let you poke and prod at them time and again. Even under the best circumstances, you have to go into every case taking as if you were never going to have this particular chance again. You will never be able to recapture this moment, to have this particular interplay with this patient again. So you must make the best of it. You and your patient must communicate fully, and then you must take all that you have learned and put it into action.

> Even under the best circumstances, you have to go into every case taking as if you were never going to have this particular chance again. . . . So you must make the best of it. You and your patient must communicate fully, and then you must take all that you have learned and put it into action.

Remember, Kent said that the case is only half cured. You have gathered the information that you need in order to act. If you can't make the right use of that information, if you don't act prudently and appropriately, then you have only done half the job. As important as case taking is, you won't get the job done unless you can organize and synthesize the information you worked so hard to gather and then put it into action in the form of a remedy.

CHAPTER FIFTEEN

Case Management

After you have finished taking the case, everything else is case management.

Case management includes the research you undertake in order to find the remedy. It includes the thinking that you put into the choice of the potency and dosage. It includes all the notes you make in your research and all the notes you take as you follow the remedy's action through your patient's reports. And it involves a statement of what you learned from your failure or success at the end of the treatment.

Many would-be practitioners want to take shortcuts in their case management. But I have found that this quite simply is not a good idea. One homeopath I knew insisted that he never had to repertorize his cases, that he took them and then, based upon the information that he had memorized over time, he selected the remedy. The fact that he had an awful track record when it came to cures never seemed to suggest to him that he try another way.

The best and most successful cases are always those that are managed well. The cure, like God, is always in the details.

Starting In

The first step in basic case management—and this will hold for the simplest acute case and the most complex chronic condition—is to work with the symptoms so that they can yield usable information.

In a simple acute case, such as a mechanical injury, this can be a relatively quick and easy procedure. There will, in the first place, usually be only a very few symptoms associated with the case. In such a case, the practitioner administers first aid—examines the wound or injury, cleans it, etc. Then all that remains is to select the remedy that best suits the patient's total symptoms associated with that injury. Just as the case taking in such an instance can be no more than a few seconds in which you examine the patient and ask a few basic questions, the remedy selection will often not involve much more than choosing between two remedies that both may be of use. In fact, this is the rare instance in which a home guide to homeopathy may be quite helpful to a successful outcome.

While the process of gathering information about the patient's unique symptoms and then using that information to choose the remedy most similar in action to those symptoms stays the same in more complex situations, the *manner* in which this selection is made gets a good deal more complicated. Where once a remedy was selected from the handful available, each of which was thoroughly known in the totality of its action, today we have to depend upon research and upon the knowledge of those homeopaths who came before us in order to have the information we need in the practice of homeopathy.

Remember, when Hahnemann was himself practicing homeopathy, he did not have the reference books at his disposal that we do today. In fact the Repertory, the book that most of us depend on every day in order to get from symptoms to remedies for those symptoms, had yet to be invented. But in that Hahnemann himself had both proven the remedies in his pharmacy and had potentized them himself by hand, he had an intimate knowledge of the full range of remedies used in all their potencies that no one today could match. In that most of us have never taken part in a clinical proving of any remedy, and in that I doubt any of us could potentize a remedy by hand even if we had a laboratory full of clean glass beakers and clean water in which to dilute and succuss our little hearts out, we are at a clear disadvantage when it comes to selecting a remedy.

In that we live in a world in which we order our remedies over the Internet—remedies that are made in factories by machines instead of being painstakingly created by hand—we are now, just by virtue of our lives and the time in which we live, a bit removed from homeopathy as Hahnemann meant it to be practiced.

Many fewer of our practitioners today have the working knowledge of the remedies than did those who practiced two hundred years ago. This most certainly is not the fault of the practitioner, since, again, they, like us are ordering their remedies from a factory and the number of remedies that have to be chosen among has grown so dramatically throughout the years. In Hahnemann's time there were only dozens of remedies available. (Remember that the early remedies, with few exceptions like Sepia, were taken from the standard herbal pharmacy of the day. These were, for the most part, medicines that came from nearby geographical regions and medicines with a known track record. Today, virtually any substance—including allopathic medicines themselves—have been potentized into homeopathic remedies.) A modern homeopath, on the other hand, quite literally has thousands of remedies to choose from, and many different potencies of each.

This can be a daunting task. Most especially when the homeopath looks at his notes and sees the huge amount of information he has gathered. This is something he is going to have to put into order before he can find the remedy.

The Symptoms

In taking the case, the homeopath has already made the distinction between the subjective and the objective symptoms—between the symptoms that either he or the caregiver have noted and the symptoms that only the patient himself can know. This is important later. After a remedy is given, it will again be important to record the patient's comments in his own words, as much as is possible, in order to ascertain the direction in which the case is moving.

But there are many other ways to work with symptoms.

First, it is important to be able to categorize each symptom, so as to best use that bit of information in order to find a cure.*

Among the different types of symptoms are as follows:

- **Chief Complaint:** I start with this one, because in working with a case, I tend to always start with this one. The Chief Complaint is the specific symptom or group of symptoms that so bothered the patient that he sought medical help. It is important to note that, in the course of treatment, this Chief Complaint may prove to be a great deal more important to the patient than it is to the practitioner in finding that curative remedy, but the simple fact that this was the problem that caused him to seek help means that it must be given some special consideration by the practitioner.

- **Common Symptoms:** These are just what you'd think they are—the symptoms that are common to most of the people who are suffering from the same complaint. They are also, therefore, the symptoms that, when researched, will yield the largest number of potential remedies. They are, therefore, not very useful at all to the practitioner in determining the remedy.

- **General Symptoms:** Although these sound as if they are similar to the common symptoms, they are, in fact, not. General Symptoms are general in that they are

---

* Note here that these various classifications of symptoms are not directly from Hahnemann. Rather, they are the work of various homeopaths since his time. Some classifications will work for you better than will others. Many, as you will find as you research this subject more, are merely different ways of saying the same thing. Sadly, homeopaths sometimes act like allopaths in thinking that if they can give something a new name that they can "own" it. The most important point about symptoms is that you are going to have to find some way of your own to weed out the important symptoms from those that, while they may be troublesome to the patient, are just not going to be that helpful to you in finding a curative remedy. This, like every other aspect of case taking and management, is very hard to put down in words on a page. This knowledge is best learned in the clinical setting.

felt within the whole of the patient's body or being. They are symptoms of the whole person. (Remember in case taking that information was sought as to the quality of each of the patient's symptoms? And remember that information was then sought about the quality of how the patient felt as a whole—what, for instance, makes the patient feel better or worse as a whole person? The answer to that question and the others pertaining to wholeness was a list of the patient's Generals.) These symptoms can be very helpful, most especially when combined with the Specific Symptoms (see next), in finding the remedy.

- **Specific Symptoms (Local Symptoms):** These are those symptoms that relate to specific parts of the patient's body or being. This could be a face that is discolored red, for instance. It can also relate to sides of the body, like a left-sided sciatica. It should be noted that, in some cases, the patient may present a group of specific symptoms that, in reality, may be considered as a whole to be a General Symptom.*

- **Determining Symptoms (Secondary Symptoms):** These are symptoms that are perhaps secondary in consideration to the Chief Complaint, but that help refine our understanding of that complaint. They are often Generals, but not always. For instance, if the Chief Complaint is a terrible cold, in which the patient has a runny nose and runny eyes as well, with a watery flow from each, and that patient has a fever and no desire for food. We can narrow down our field of possible remedies if we can also know at what time of day or night the patient's symptoms are worse or better, what the patient's pattern of the symptoms is. The patient who feels much worse around midnight suggests one course of treatment. The patient who is worse first thing in the morning suggests another.

- **Concomitant Symptoms:** These are the symptoms that occur at the same time, most often as part of the Chief Complaint. They may be in any area of the being, although, most often, you will find them in the same part of the body. Examples would be swollen, runny eyes and raw, sore throat occurring together in allergies or a headache that occurs at the same time as diarrhea during flu.

- **Alternating Symptoms:** These are similar to Concomitant Symptoms. In this case, the symptoms simply alternate. First comes the headache, then comes the diarrhea. If you can determine that this is the pattern in a given illness that a patient is

---

* This is a really good tip: The best way to tell a patient's Generals from his Specifics is often couched in the patient's own language. If the patient refers to a symptom with "I have," such as "I have a pain in my left side," that may be considered a Specific symptom. If the patient, on the other hand, refers to the symptom with "I am," he is giving you the information that the symptom affects every part of him. Therefore, "I am unable to sleep," or "I feel better outside," are both examples of General Symptoms.

experiencing, then this patterning, like that of the Concomitants, can be helpful in finding the correct remedy.

- **Characteristic Symptoms:** These symptoms can be very helpful in narrowing down the field of possible remedies. These are the symptoms that are unique to this particular patient's experience of his disease. If, for instance, you have a patient with a terribly upset stomach, who has been vomiting perhaps, but who presents a perfectly clean tongue, you have a symptom that will help lead you to a remedy.

- **Keynote Symptoms:** Keynotes are the next step toward truly peculiar. Where the Characteristic Symptoms show the way in which the patient is "personalizing" his disease, the Keynotes are the true oddities. These are the little facts—like the fact that the Phosphorus patient* can be so easily nauseated that they cannot bear to wash the dishes because they become ill if they submerge their hands in water— that can lead right to a remedy. Beware the Keynotes, however. I have known practitioners who prescribed by the Keynotes alone, thinking that to be a really clever shortcut to treatment. It is not. Keynotes, like every other sort of symptom, have to be placed within the context of the whole case.

These are the general classifications of symptoms. With these classifications, it is possible to organize a "family tree" of the case. This places the Chief Complaint at the root of the tree, and all symptoms associated with that complaint, that define and refine it as it is being experienced by a particular patient, branch off from there. It might be helpful to quite literally make an illustration of the case using this sort of format. Or it might also be helpful to organize the case using 3 X 5 cards, and color-coding them by type of symptom. Or this may all be a bit anal for you and you may want to just list the symptoms on a legal pad or computer screen. In any case, by first zero-

---

* The use of the term "Phosphorus patient" is something of a shorthand. More completely stated, it should read "the patient for whom the remedy Phosphorus is the indicated remedy." In homeopathic jargon, however, we will shorten that to the simpler "Phosphorus patient." In fact, you will find that homeopaths most often will refer to patients with the name of the remedy that is most similar to them. As in "he's a real Sulphur" or "she's a true Natrum Mur," that sort of thing. It's easier. As we said, in Chapter 4, in homeopathic jargon, practitioners make use of what is called the "drug diagnosis." Where allopaths exclusively use a disease diagnosis, by which they refer to the case by the name of the disease that is being treated, homeopaths use a "drug diagnosis." In a "drug diagnosis," the practitioner does not refer to the patient by their disease—in fact, some classical homeopaths believe that it is best never to give a specific group of symptoms a name, as that name implies both a map or treatment and a potential outcome or rate of success for that treatment—but instead by the name of the remedy that, in the full sphere of its action, most clearly mirrors the full range of symptoms that the patient is experiencing.

ing in on the Chief Complaint, and then by going to the Secondary Symptoms that refine it, and the Keynotes that further narrow it, you can get a good idea of just what is going on.

Refining Symptoms

Now that the symptoms have been listed and organized and you have an idea of what the case is about, it is important that the symptoms be further refined. In order to do this, you must turn again to the case as the patient revealed it.

In order to refine the symptoms, we have to separate them out into individual parts. About each individual symptom, we need to know the following:

- Sensation: How do his symptoms feel, exactly? Does the patient's headache have a burning sensation, or does it feel as if someone were driving a nail into his head?

- Location: Exactly where is this symptom located? Is it a headache in the forehead or on top of the head, or does it cover the entire head?

- Duration: How long has this symptom been in place? And in what order did it appear, when compared with the patient's other symptoms?

- Onset: Find out about the circumstances surrounding the beginning of this symptom. When did the patient first notice it? What was he doing, smelling, eating, or drinking at the time? Under what circumstances did the symptom begin?

- Modality: I find this to be the most useful modifier of symptoms. When we learn the modalities of the symptoms, we are finding out what makes them feel better or worse. The headache that requires an icepack requires a treatment different from the headache that requires a hot shower. In tracing the modalities, we are tracing the patient's instincts. What does he want to do in order to make that symptom feel better and what makes it feel worse? This is very important information.

After you have gathered this modifying information concerning each individual symptom, then look to your General Symptoms. Try to ascertain the same information about the patient as a whole—most especially the modalities that relate to him as a whole being. Can he not bear to be in a warm room? That is some good information to know. Does he insist on being covered up and will allow not a single bit of air to move in the room, because he is so very cold? Get out the Nux Vomica.

As you refine the remedies, add this information to your family tree. You are now getting a clearer and clearer image of your case, with a defined Chief Complaint, supporting Secondary Symptoms, and modifying information about each. If you can avoid letting that family tree turn into a forest, you are moving in the right direction.

Hekla Lava

What must be avoided is getting trapped in the forest of the case because there are so many trees.

As Kent taught, many beginning homeopaths know only a handful of remedies and use them almost exclusively and have about an 80 percent rate of cure. As they study more, take more classes; they learn more and more remedies. Soon they know of hundreds of remedies, and how to find out about hundreds more if they think they need them. They start using hundreds of different remedies, taking pride in the fact that they know all about Hekla Lava.*

So they give many different, increasingly exotic remedies to their patients and they have a cure rate of about 40 percent, but everyone is certainly very impressed with their apparent knowledge of homeopathy.

After many years of study, the practitioner now knows a great deal about homeopathy. He has studied many different remedies in their actions, and he has the practical, clinical knowledge of homeopathy to match his philosophical zeal.

In the end, he again mostly uses that handful of remedies that he first learned, Arnica, Sulphur, Natrum Muriaticum, Rhus Toxicodendron, Sepia, Lachesis, Phosphorus, Lycopodium, Aconite, Pulsatilla and the like, and he has a success rate of about 90 percent.

This is a wise warning from Kent. Our very desire to get everything right, to fully understand every aspect of a case can so often not only confuse everything in a muddle of facts, remedies and symptoms, but can actually make it incurable, if the confusion of remedies leads to a confusion of treatments.

As a general rule of thumb, I have found that a generally healthy person who happens, at the moment to, be sick, will likely need one of our major remedies, the so-called polycrests.† (see page 144) It is the patient who is very, very sick—who, for instance, is suffering a breakdown of his immune system—who

> As a general rule of thumb . . . a generally healthy person who happens, at the moment, to be sick, will likely need one of our major remedies, the so-called polycrests. It is the patient who is very, very sick . . . who will begin to require the very small, very rare little remedies as a common occurrence.

will begin to require the very small, very rare little remedies as a common occurrence. This is not to say that we never make use of the smaller remedies in the day-to-day practice of homeopathy, only that if we abandon logic and common sense in the name

---

* The remedy Hekla Lava is made from the volcanic ash taken from Mt. Hekla in Iceland. Good for cases involving tennis elbow, all other aspects of the case matching, of course.

of a "complete" case taking (which, in reality, can become an overblown mess if we gather so much unnecessary information that we can't separate out what will actually guide us to a remedy from what will not) then we are going to do little good for the patient, which is the whole point of homeopathic practice.

Again, in case management, as in case taking, the management must suit the case. Which is another argument for the fact that no one studying or practicing homeopathy should ever work beyond his or her skill level. If you have a really good grasp of acute cases, a real feel for how they happen and how best they can be treated, then, by all means, concentrate on acute cases. And, in doing so, you will do a great deal of good. (After all, can the most skilled allopath actually treat a cold and help his patient to recover more quickly and, in doing so, help strengthen that patient against the next oncoming cold? Acute treatments can work miracles.)

It is also important to note that Kent's injunction would suggest that you should also, whenever possible, stick to the remedies you know. By that, I do not suggest that, in a case needing Nux Vomica, you give the patient Arnica, because you are more

---

† (from page 143) These are the remedies that, through clinical use, have proven to not only have a wide number range of uses, but have also shown themselves to have impact on many parts of a patient's being, body, mind, and emotions. Because of this, they are the remedies most used, and, therefore, responsible for the most cures. Beginning practitioners would do well to first study these.

These polycrest remedies are also the templates for what are known as "constitutional types." In that these remedies have been fully mapped in their actions, they have all shown an impact reaching beyond mere physical symptoms to identified and fully described mental, emotional, spiritual and behavioral symptoms. Within their sphere of actions they, therefore, give portraits of fully rounded human beings. Some homeopaths practicing constitutional medicine see the long-term patterning of a patient's symptoms as mirroring one of these remedies, they consider that patient to be of a particular constitutional type. The idea is that all of us, as we are beset by illness, trauma—either physical or emotional—and life circumstances, become locked into a particular pattern of living in order to best survive. These survival patterns can last for many years, until we either find a better adaptation, leading to better health, or decline into a weaker state of being. Throughout our lives we can pile up several layers, each defined by particular circumstances and particular symptoms of response to those circumstances. It is therefore the purpose of constitutional homeopathy to move us back through these layers, releasing the symptoms that are still suppressed within. As the layer is released, the symptoms are removed and the patient moves nearer to a state of perfect health.

It must be noted here that even though the concept of constitutional types helps the homeopath to identify how the patient has in the past responded to his or her life, and gives a remedy name to the group of patients who, in similar circumstances have reacted in the same way, it does not necessarily give indication of present treatment. In other words, it may be a fairly simple matter to come to understand that an angry, type-A male patient is likely of the Nux Vomica constitutional type, but that does not mean that he may need the remedy Nux at the given moment. Only through case taking can the indicated remedy be found, even if the constitutional type may be screaming to make itself known.

familiar with that remedy. No, I suggest that, before you treat anyone, you must become very familiar with the remedies themselves. You must study before you start handing out remedies, to yourself or anyone else. So, if you have studied well the remedies that are most often associated with mechanical injuries—Arnica, Rhus, Bellis Perennis, and the like—then you should also, until you learn more about homeopathy, stick to cases that involve simple mechanical injuries as well.

Never let your own pride keep you from seeking professional help when needed. Just as I have always stayed quite conservative about actually taking or giving remedies, I have always remained quite conservative about the cases that I choose to take. Especially today, when the woods are filled with practitioners, we should never hesitate to ask for help. In doing so, we might learn something more about homeopathy that will allow us to be able to actually treat the next case ourselves.

The Three-Legged Stool

Hahnemann gave some great advice concerning complicated cases. And certainly today we are seeing more and more complicated cases. As the psora (the miasm largely responsible for functional disorders of all sorts) piles up generation after generation, more and more of us are chronically ill, and ill with more than one chronic complaint at a time. In allopathic medicine, this has lead to a generation of patients who take a dozen or more medicines daily, each one for some other aspect of their complaints. In homeopathic cases, this leads to case taking that can be so complex that it takes hours to unfold, leaving many pages of information on the case, from symptoms to case histories to family medical histories.

In these cases, it is hard to know what to do. After all, how can you fully structure a case that has a dozen or more symptoms? How can you organize all that information and then modify the symptoms as well? When there is not one Chief Complaint, but twenty, what do you do?

Hahnemann suggests that we consider the three-legged stool. Just as this little piece of furniture is the sturdiest of structures, so, too, does it represent a way of looking at a case that can be helpful in finding a cure.

When faced with a case that is cluttered with symptoms, start out not by looking at the details, but by looking at the whole. Then see if you can isolate three central issues. (I don't suggest that you must always choose exactly three, but look at what is going on in the case, try to identify the Chief Complaint and then identify the secondary issues.* [see page 146]) Then move from general specific. Take those issues apart; look at what symptoms flow through those issues, and what patterns exist that link those symptoms.

Working with a case can become all but impossible if, from the start, you find yourself in a maze of details. By starting with the whole and then moving down, always from more general to more specific, you will have, in the end, a much better understanding of the case.

The same is true in dealing with the symptoms themselves. Case management always works best if, in repertorizing the case, you always start with the General Symptoms, and then move from there down to the Chief Complaint, and from there down to Secondary Symptoms, and from there downward, from the symptoms that affect the whole of the patient's being down to the symptoms that impact upon organs or systems in the patient's body, down to the very small, specific, or peculiar symptoms.†

Unlike allopathy, homeopathy is ever a blend of the objective and the subjective, and of the detail and the whole. The homeopath that locks himself into the consideration of the details of a particular case, without also concerning himself with the generals is likely to overlook the obvious in terms of treatment.

In the same way, when dealing with a complex case that is filled with the details of many different complaints, it is important to make a judgment as to what the case is about, organizing the case so that it flows from general to specific, all in preparation of the repertorization process.

Repertorization

After the case has been organized, it is at last time to move toward the selection of the remedy. This selection process is made possible through the use of two reference books, the Repertory and the Materia Medica.

The Repertory is the tool that allows the practitioner to take all the pieces of

---

* (from page 145) In aphorism #153 of his *Organon*, Hahnemann writes, "In the search for a homeopathically specific remedy, that is, in the comparison of the complex of the natural disease's signs with the symptom sets of available medicines . . . the more *striking, exceptional, unusual, and odd* (characteristic) signs and symptoms of the disease case are to be especially and almost solely kept in view. *These, above all, must correspond to very similar ones in the set of the medicine sought* if it is to be the most fitting one for cure. The more common and indeterminate symptoms (a lack of appetite, headache, lassitude, restless sleep, discomfort, etc.) are to be seen with almost every disease and medicine and thus deserve little attention unless they are more closely characterized." With this Hahnemann helps us build our three-legged stool. By staying with the unusual symptoms and thoroughly investigating both the symptoms and the remedies that can create that unusual symptom, cases can be narrowed in their focus and, more important, clarified in terms of treatment.

† In fact, as we shall see ahead, in repertorizing the case, the practitioner may choose to not, even at first, repertorize the Keynote or Peculiar Symptoms. But whether they are repertorized early on or not, the Keynotes should be checked only at the end of research, and used as a means of verifying the selected remedy, and not as a tool to its selection. This is the safest and correct use of the Keynote symptoms.

information that they have gathered and organized concerning a particular case, and translate them into the names of a handful of remedies, each of which has the potential for curing the case.

The Repertory is a book that contains all the information that has been gathered in the clinical provings of remedies. It lists all the symptoms, from the most general to the most peculiar or specific, that have been shown to be created through the use of homeopathic remedies.*

It may be said, therefore, that the Repertory has replaced the firsthand experience of homeopathic drugs and their specific actions that Hahnemann and the other founding fathers of homeopathy had stored in their own brains. Truly, in today's world, we could not successfully practice homeopathy without our Repertories.

Is this to say that a Repertory is always needed in order to select the remedy for a given case? No. Certainly there are those cases, household emergencies mostly, that are so simple that no one need run for the Repertory. The case is taken with a quick examination and by asking a few questions. Then, based on rudimentary knowledge of homeopathy, a remedy is selected. Or a skilled homeopath may well immediately know the remedy that will be needed in a given case without needing to repertorize. But the rule of thumb is that the case will need to be thoroughly repertorized, which is to say that each symptom will have to be considered in terms of the *rubrics* in the Repertory that speak to that symptom. Rubrics are the individual listings in the Repertory. They may be quite general in nature, in which case they may reference a large number of remedies, each of which, to a greater or lesser degree, will be effective in treating that symptom. The rubrics list the symptoms in three degrees of import, in normal, italic, and boldface print. The lowest level, in normal print, suggests remedies that, although they did appear in some cases of clinical proving, are not considered as strong contenders for the symptom. As the print moves from *italic* to **boldface**, the remedies listed become more and more important to the symptom under consideration.

Repertorization can be a humbling task, in that it can take hours to work through and in that it requires the homeopath—be he young or old, skilled or unskilled—to write out the rubrics under consideration and the remedies suggested by each. Even in

---

* Perhaps I overstate here. There is no such a thing as a "master" Repertory, one that contains all knowledge of symptoms. Instead, there are several available on the market, each of which is the work of a single author or group of authors. Each, to the best of its ability, lists the symptoms experienced by patients and the remedies that have been found effective for those symptoms. But *no* Repertory should be considered perfect or exhaustive. In fact, you will often find written the margins of the pages of a given homeopath's Repertory the names of the remedies that should have been included for a specific symptom. See Chapter 17 for more information on Repertories and Materia Medicas.

this age of computer programs and other aids to repertorization, I consider it of great importance that each repertorization be written out by hand, and by the same hand that will ultimately make the prescription. This is because, in the process of looking it up and writing it out, something strange can happen—the essence of the case can begin to become apparent to the person repertorizing. During that long process, the practitioner is, in some strange way, spending time getting to know his patient, and getting to understand him. No computer can give you the insights into a case that the simple, if grueling, task of repertorization can. For this reason, many skilled homeopaths, even if they feel strongly about a remedy based upon the initial case taking, will still get down the Repertory and get started in their research.

In repertorizing, it is important that the practitioner make use of the right rubrics, and only of rubrics that actually accurately describe some aspect of the case. The case can be well taken, and well organized, but if the repertorization is based on the wrong rubrics, then it can be quite impossible to find the right remedy. Therefore, as with anything else, hard work will be required in learning to use the Repertory. Any rubric that is at all questionable in terms of its direct description of a symptom should not be considered. It would be better to base a prescription on a dozen rubrics that are well chosen, then to base it on a hundred that do not all speak to the case.

Anyone unfamiliar with his or her Repertory will find it of little use during a medical emergency. A new student of homeopathy should, before ever turning to the Repertory in a time of need, study it well in a time of calm.

Finally, in repertorizing a case, as in organizing it, one should begin with the General Symptoms and work down from there. The General rubrics, while long and involved, will list remedies that may not appear in the smaller, more specific rubrics. And as no Repertory is perfect, there may be gaps in the smaller rubrics that are filled in by the larger. In using only the smallest possible rubrics that list the fewest number of remedies, and, thereby, saving wear and tear on their hands and wrists, unskilled homeopaths seek yet another shortcut with which they can court disaster.

Materia Medica

While the Repertory is an important tool in the selection of a remedy, the Materia Medica is the very heart of homeopathic study. Each homeopathic Materia Medica contains an exhaustive listing of the efficacy of each individual remedy, listed alphabetically. As each Materia Medica is the work of an individual homeopath, they differ in some material, but each represents the life's work of a practitioner who dedicated his life to the understanding of homeopathy. Therefore, each Materia Medica is a unique gift, and each offers valuable insights into the remedies and their uses.

So, while the Repertory may be an important tool, one that allows the practitioner to narrow down their choice of a remedy from thousands to perhaps three or four (it is very rare for a remedy to so stand out in repertorization that the practitioner can be sure that it is the absolute best remedy for the patient), it is the Materia Medica that is always the final word on the case. We research with the Repertory, but prescribe from the Materia Medica.

> **We research with the Repertory, but prescribe from the Materia Medica.**

This means that, after all the case taking and organization and repertorization, we are not done yet. After the remedies have been narrowed down by the simple mathematics of some appearing more often, or in a more prominent manner, than do others in the process of repertorization, it is time to put the pad and pencils and Repertory aside. At this point, unless there is some pressing emergency, I find it best to walk away from the process for a time. When I return, I pick up the Materia Medica and look again at the listings for each of the remedies that seem possible for the case. I may read the listing in several different Materia Medicas in order to get a full range of descriptions and opinions.

At this point, I no longer think of a patient in terms of his individual symptoms and their peculiarities. I am now considering the patient as a whole being. Just as it is important, in considering a case, to be able to break that case down into its details, it is also important to be able to look at it whole. In this final process, I consider that whole being and try, with the Materia Medica, to match that whole patient to the whole action of a remedy. The best match will result in the best cure—that you can always depend on.

If it comes down to two remedies and I cannot choose, then I again go back to the details and check them in the Materia Medica (beware, however, that the Materia Medica is not nearly as specific in details as is the Repertory—the fact that some small symptom is not listed in the Materia Medica does not mean that the remedy in question cannot be effective in treating it) and then return again to the patient as a whole. The remedy that, on balance, speaks to the details and to the wholeness of the case will be my remedy of choice.

I wish I could say that, at the end of this process, you will always be sure of your choice, or that you will always make the right choice. The only thing that I can say is that, with a lot of work and with an ever-increasing amount of experience (good or bad, successful or not) to call upon, your chances of making the right choice will increase.

But even when you have done everything you can, even when you give the remedy with a great sense of security in the amount of work you have done and the quality of that work, sometimes the best choice remedy will simply not work, or will work for a short time and then fail. In these cases, you have no choice but to follow up, to start again, and to work even harder next time.

Selecting Potency and Dosage

Another potential pitfall of homeopathic treatment has to do with potency and dosage. Just as you can do everything right and then choose the wrong rubrics to ruin the case, you can also choose the right rubrics, select the right remedy, and then ruin the case by choosing the wrong potency or by giving the wrong number of doses.*

The best way to approach both is to be as conservative as possible. This is especially the case with elderly or chronically ill patients. These cases involve a weakened vital force, and that vital force does not need you shoving it around in a feeble attempt to make things better. I believe that it is always better to start slowly and simply in homeopathic treatments.

That means that I always start with a single dose of any medicine.

Then I remember something that S. K. Bannerjea, my first teacher, taught me: "The Three Ws."

Simply put, these mean Wait + Watch = Wisdom. Give the dose, and then do nothing. Wait. Watch for the changes in the patient, in his demeanor, his energy, his symptoms. Then, based on the changes that you see (or lack thereof), consider the remedy, the potency, and the dose once more in the context of what you have witnessed. Is that remedy, based upon all that you've seen, the best possible choice in its present rate of potency and dose?

As a rule of thumb, the weaker the vital force, the lower the potency you want to use to start the case. You can always give the remedy again at a future point in a higher potency if the remedy proves correct, but the potency is not great enough to finish the case. But, if you stir things up too quickly, aggravations may result, and, in the case of a weakened patient, an aggravation can be an uncomfortable or even a dangerous thing.

And, of course, we never want to begin a case with multiple doses. We don't want to create any possibility of a proving, in which case it may become difficult to know if the symptoms are a continuation of the natural symptoms, or symptoms that have been artificially grafted on the patient by the remedy itself.

So move carefully with both potency and dose, remembering that, in homeopathic cure, we are always to do the least amount possible to create a cure.

The Impact of the Dose

Once the remedy has been given, then there are only a limited number of things that

---

* At times the sheer amount of work involved and the myriad ways in which you can screw up a case may make you wish you had never gotten involved in homeopathy. But then you will one day give a remedy that changes someone's life, or gives them back their life, and then everything seems worth it.

can happen. In some cases, the patient will feel much better. In other cases, he will feel worse. And, sometimes, nothing at all will happen.

An improvement can come in many different forms, however. Typically, a patient who has been given a well-selected remedy in a reasonable potency and dose will react with an increase in energy. They will feel better as a whole being. Now, this may not always mean that their symptoms will go away immediately. The headache, cold, or other malady may not change right away. Instead, the patient will typically report that, although they still have their headache, they are better able to cope with it. That their symptoms do not bother them as much as they did before. If this happens, or if the patient shows a literal increase in energy by moving around more and more freely than before, you can be sure that the cure has begun.

In the same way, sleep can be a wonderful sign of improvement. If the patient falls into a restful and peaceful sleep after having been given their remedy, then you can be sure that they will awaken feeling better.

In some cases, the patient will report an immediate change in a symptom or a group of symptoms. This change can be for the better or the worse. But the fact that a change has occurred in the symptoms, which research has told you the selected remedy has the power to affect, indicates that this remedy will do some good.

Certainly, from the patient's perspective at least, an improvement of symptoms, or the disappearance of same, is the preferred route to cure. But a temporary increase in symptoms, that which is called an *aggravation*, may also indicate that the case is on its way to being cured. In fact, in the treatment of acute illnesses, it is quite common and perhaps unavoidable that a brief aggravation occurs as the remedy begins its work. The patient who, minutes after taking his remedy, has a worse sore throat than he did before needs to be assured that the remedy will soon bring about a cure.

If an aggravation is not brief, if it does not fade in a matter of hours, or if the aggravation is overwhelming to the patient, then the practitioner must stop and reassess the case. Such an aggravation may indicate that the remedy given was in too high a potency for the patient's vital force to deal with. In this case, it may be necessary to blunt the action of the remedy by antidoting it with another remedy—Nux Vomica is commonly used to antidote the impact of other remedies—or with known homeopathic antidotes like coffee.* (see page 152)

Simple aggravations—those that are caused by a single dose of a remedy and that do not too greatly tax the patient—will fade in a matter of hours, taking with them many of the symptoms of the original illness.

Remember, if some change occurs, it is necessary to follow the progress of the change before taking any other action. If the aggravation fades and improvement begins, or if the case simply moves from the dose to improvement, it is important that the remedy not be repeated or replaced with another remedy as long as the improvement continues. All homeopathic remedies are given on the basis of need. As long as another dose is not needed, it should never be given. Those who prescribe by telling their patients to take the remedy every three hours, or who give one more dose "for the road" are practicing allopathic medicine.

Now, if that third possibility occurs, and nothing whatsoever happens, the first thing to do is nothing. Sometimes, in their great desire to help the patient, the practitioner will make the mistake of giving the next dose—either or a new remedy or the old again in a greater potency—when, if they had only waited a bit, the first dose would have worked brilliantly. So give the remedy a chance. Check with the Materia Medica to see how quickly the selected remedy is known to work. Some, like the mineral-based remedies Silicea and Graphities, may work more slowly than do others. In the same way, some remedies work better in repeated doses than do others. It is always a good idea to check on the specifics of a remedy before giving it.

The Second Prescription

Sometimes the first remedy used will complete the task of cure, sometimes it will not. Sometimes the practitioner will be called upon to solve a riddle—a well-selected remedy has not worked at all, or has done some good but not completed the cure. The practitioner then has to decide what to do. Should he give a new remedy to the patient with the hopes that it will work? Or should he give the same remedy in a different potency, with the hopes that that was all that was needed, an adjustment of the original remedy? Or should he do nothing and wait and see what happens?

There is no set answer. But in all instances, the practitioner is called upon to reconsider both his case taking and his research of the case. He has to be sure that he was working from sufficient information upon which to base his prescription and that, in repertorizing the case, he chose the right rubrics and interpreted them correctly. This may also involve again studying his Materia Medica for insights into the remedies themselves.

---

* (from page 151) Antidotes are medical substances whose power it is to interfere with the working of remedies. Coffee is a known antidote, but, in my opinion, it only works for people who don't regularly drink coffee, and for whom it is a powerful stimulant. But during homeopathic treatment, sensitive people may have to avoid coffee and other strong stimulants and smell. Perfume can antidote some people. And Hahnemann was known to carry spirits of camphor with him. He would have his patients sniff the camphor if the effects of the remedy given proved to be too strong.

I'm not too much a believer in antidotes, since experience tells me that people who drink coffee daily will not antidote with coffee—in fact, you could give them their remedy in coffee and it would work just fine. But just as some practitioners practice by aggravations, they also practice using coffee to antidote their aggravations. It all seems like sloppy work to me. If you would give the right potency and dosage to begin with, you wouldn't have to always be undoing what you have done.

As difficult as the original prescription may be, the second prescription is worse still. Even if the case is going just fine up until then, it can be very difficult to know just when to make a change in a remedy or its potency. Actually, it is easier to know what to do when your first attempt at a remedy was a flop, than it was when the first remedy worked fine but failed to complete the cure.*

Only by going over the case again and again can the practitioner move forward with a sense that he is doing what is right.

Following Up

Certainly whether the first remedy was successful or not, it is important that the practitioner follow up with his patient. In that they are joint partners in the patient's cure, it is vital that the communication established between them continue throughout the entire process of treatment.

The gathering of both the subjective and objective symptoms is an ongoing process. This means that, if the healing team involved in the case does not include a very trustworthy caretaker, the practitioner will need to follow up with this patient in person, so that he may himself examine the patient. If an attentive caretaker oversees the doses of the remedies, as well as the diet and environment of the patient, then follow-ups may sometimes take place via the telephone or email.

As long as the essential communication occurs, the method by which it takes place is not important. What is important is that no second prescription be made unless and until both patient and practitioner are satisfied that it is being made on the basis of a full understanding of what has taken place from the initial treatment.

Learning from Success, Learning from Failure

There is no such thing as an all-knowing homeopath. No one gets it right all the time. But there is much that each practitioner can learn, both from his successes and his failures. And, honestly, I believe that most practitioners would admit that they have learned much more from their failures than from their successes. You only have to see a patient experience the discomfort of a severe aggravation once in order to be much more careful in the future not to give any remedy in too high an initial potency. In the same way, a few experiences in sloppy repertorization will induce most of us to either spend more hours in working with the text or go out and find a school in which we can learn the art of researching remedies.

There is no disgrace in failure, as long as the patient does not ultimately suffer

---

* It should also be noted that irregularities in the patient's diet or toxins in his environment may both interfere with the working of the remedy. And, if the patient fails to take his remedy, I can guarantee that it will not work for him. These things must also be considered in any reassessment of the case.

from our failures. As long as the practitioner knows when to admit defeat and ask for help or when to simply help the patient to get to a better skilled practitioner, then there is no reason for that practitioner to do anything other than to try harder next time. In truth, homeopathy is not a calling for the proud. If you cannot humble yourself enough to work not for your own glory, but solely for the good of the patient, then you have no business here.

> There is no such thing as an all-knowing homeopath. No one gets it right all the time. But there is much that each practitioner can learn, both from his successes and his failures.

As for learning, a good bit of it will depend upon the care with which you have taken the case, organized it, and researched it. It also depends upon how carefully you have taken notes on the case itself and how it unfolded from first to last. In reviewing excellent notes, a great deal may be learned that can be put to even better use in the next case. Those who do not bother to take careful notes will find themselves with no lessons learned.

I find that it also helps to always close the case with a review of it. I like to write about the case, from start to finish, how I saw it at first and how it turned out to be. If I saw one sort of remedy, but another was actually successful, I note this. If I allowed myself to think one way, ignoring the facts of the case, or something that was right in front of my nose, I note that as well. And, of course, if I got the whole thing right and experienced a great success, then I write about that at great length.

If there is something to take away from this chapter it is the simple fact that case management, like case taking, is a serious thing. It is a great deal of work. It can be a thankless thing as well, as a successful remedy is the very thing that the patient expects from the very beginning. The fact that your treatment worked so well may not come as any surprise to the patient. It may not be anything that they think is worth thanking you over.

In a very real way, the work itself is the reward. The hard work is not the thing that we just have to accept if we are going to be homeopaths—it is the very reason that we are homeopaths.

Homeopaths are the rarest of practitioners. To be effective, they must be open enough to witness their patients just as they are. They must be willing to see and understand and never judge. They must also have minds that allow them to work almost simultaneously in seeing great detail and in ignoring all details and seeing only the whole. They have to be willing to work when others are sleeping, hunching over their Repertories at their kitchen tables, while the house is silent and the shadows are deep.

CHAPTER SIXTEEN

Animal/Vegetable/Mineral

One way of learning how best to use homeopathic remedies is to consider the actual physical source of those remedies. Anything can be made into a homeopathic remedy. Any natural substance—animal, vegetable, or mineral—can be made into a remedy. Man-made substances and objects as well can be potentized into homeopathic form, as can your own tissue, from hair to blood to urine. Each, when potentized, will reveal its range of activities. Some can be quite surprising. A remedy taken from a powerfully medicinal substance may turn out to be a very narrow or shallow remedy, while a remedy taken from a very benign substance—Natrum Muriaticum, taken from ordinary table salt is a good example of this—can become a very powerful medicine.

There's a story concerning Hahnemann that illustrates this. Like all stories concerning Hahnemann, I cannot vouch for its complete historical truth, I can only say that, since it illustrates my point so nicely, I cannot help but mention it here.

Samuel Hahnemann was once treating a patient who was proving very difficult to cure. When the remedies that first came to mind for the case failed to lead to a cure Hahnemann did what he always would do and inspected the man's personal environments. Where he lived and where he worked.*

While the man's home environment proved perfectly healthful, his work environment was more interesting in terms of possible causes for the man's illness. As he always did, Hahnemann asked the man to just go about his business and carefully

---

* This is just as good an idea today as it was in Hahnemann's time. Just as he learned a great deal about his patient's health by witnessing his environment, so we can make the same judgments today. Many aspects of our environment—from carpets and lighting to dampness and smells—can determine our health just as how we store our remedies can determine their potency. Remedies that are stored on top of the television set cannot be counted on to keep good potency—electromagnetic fields of all sorts should be avoided, as energy interferes with energy.

watched how he interacted with the environment. Now this particular patient was an artist. He would tint pictures using the squid ink that, to this day, gives sepia tone its name. Hahnemann noticed that the man would first dip his brush into the ink and then, habitually, would touch the brush to the tip of his tongue before applying it to the picture. Hahnemann asked the man if he could take a little of the ink that the man was using.

He made that squid ink into a remedy and gave it to the man. As it was the source of the poisoning that lead to the man's illness, it was pure homeopathy to take that substance, potentize it, and then use it to cure the illness it had caused. It worked and the man was soon well.

In later proving his remedy, Hahnemann was no doubt astounded to find that, far from just having the ability to cleanse the body of the toxins that the substance had left, the remedy, now called Sepia, was a powerful homeopathic medicine with many uses.

Today, Sepia is one of our leading polycrests. In constitutional use, Sepia is often considered a woman's remedy, one that can be very helpful during menopause. It can also be extremely useful after pregnancy or miscarriage. Its action is wide and diverse. Among the clinical listings for the remedy are cystitis, eczema, jaundice, nosebleeds, herpes, and toothache.

So, while there is no predicting exactly what a substance will be capable of doing when it is made into a homeopathic, all remedies will have some aspects in common depending upon their source materials.

Animal, Vegetable, and Mineral

To make a gross generalization, it may be said that remedies that are taken from vegetable materials tend to be the most gentle and benign of homeopathics. These are the remedies that tend to work most quickly and are tolerated by the greatest number of patients with the least amount of aggravation.

Remedies taken from animal substances, on the other hand, tend to be the most violent—if such a word can ever actually be used when speaking of homeopathic remedies, which are never violent in the same way that allopathics are—in their action. Animal-based remedies will tend to create more aggravations than will the vegetable-based remedies. This is especially true of the venoms, remedies that are taken from snake or spider venoms. Chief among these is the polycrest Lachesis, which can be a powerful tool for patients with such conditions as hypertension and hemorrhages of all sorts. But Lachesis is a remedy that can stir up a patient's symptoms as it stirs up the vital force. This is a remedy that can cause some graphic and wild dreams, for instance, especially when first used. It is a remedy that some sensitive patients simply will not be able to tolerate. (In that Sepia is taken from squid ink and not from venom, it does not shake the tree as strongly as does Lachesis when it is first given, but even Sepia may not be well tolerated by very sensitive patients.)

There may well be cases in which it is good to remember this general rule of action that separates the vegetable from the animal remedies. In some cases, if repertorization reveals two different remedies that each are potential catalysts for the case, and one is an animal remedy, the other a vegetable, if the patient needing the remedy is weakened or sensitive, it may be best to start with the vegetable remedy and go from there.

Now the remedies that are taken from minerals tend—again, this is a gross exaggeration, and there are exceptions to the rule in every category—to work more deeply than do either the animal or vegetable remedies. They, as a group, work more slowly as well. Silicea, taken from the substance silica which comprises much of the Earth's crust, can be very slow to work, but it works very deeply, building the patient's energy reserves, his capacity to digest and to take nutrients from what he digests, and his capacity to stand strong emotionally, gaining mental, emotional, and physical strength as the remedy does its slow work.

Not all mineral remedies are slow acting to be sure. Two of our most important mineral-based remedies, Sulphur and Phosphorus, can work very quickly and very deeply as well. All three remedies, Silicea, Sulphur, and Phosphorus are true polycrests. They have the power to impact literally every cell in the human body as they bring about a cure.*

Mineral remedies as a group are especially good at building a patient's vital force, and, thereby, in generally strengthening and building endurance and energy. Further, they also tend to be especially good for the skin, and for patients with chronic diseases of the skin.

A subset of the mineral remedies contains those that are taken from metals. Because it is the common attribute of metals to conduct energy, it may be said that these metal-based remedies—gold, platinum, and silver among them—also are helpful in freeing the vital force of any blocks and in allowing the free-flow of energy throughout the body.

In that metals can come in several forms, including oxides and salts (many metal-based remedies made it into the Materia Medica in the form of their salts—chief among these are the many different Kali, or potassium-based remedies), they include

---

* A branch of what could broadly be called homeopathy is lithotherapy, or rock therapy. It is the creation of French homeopath Max Tetau. In lithotherapy, very low potencies of homeopathic remedies—all made from specific rocks like obsidian and azurite—are given to patients to combat specific diseases. Azurite, for instance, is used to treat hypertension. As with lithotherapy, we are again treating diseases and not patients, we are again in one of those shadow realms that exist around the corners of homeopathic medicine.

such substances as antimony, which harkens back to the work of the alchemists in centuries past and to Paracelsus, the great madman-healer of the sixteenth century.

Because of this, in some schools of homeopathic thought, the metal-based remedies may be seen as something special, something more transformational in terms of their healing virtue.

Nosodes

Students of homeopathy may assume that all homeopathic medicines are potentized from the very highest—and, therefore, healthiest—sources. But this is not always the case. Some specific remedies have been taken from materials that are known to be tainted or diseased. This is in keeping with the homeopathic tenant that tells us, "The stronger the poison, the stronger the cure." Just as the poisonous mineral arsenic becomes the powerful medicine Arsenicum Album, and the toxic venom of the bushmaster becomes Lachesis, so, too, do many different diseased tissues become heroic medicines.

> Just as the poisonous mineral arsenic becomes the powerful medicine Arsenicum Album, and the toxic venom of the bushmaster becomes Lachesis, so, too, do many different diseased tissues become heroic medicines.

Nosodes are the homeopathic medicines that are made from disease products.

These products may be vegetable in nature. Examples of this are the remedy Secale, a very powerful remedy that is taken from the fungus ergot that grows as black, hornlike spurs on the rye plant and Nectrianinum, which is made from a cancerous parasite that grows on trees.

More common are the nosodes that are taken from animal materials. An example of this is the remedy Ambra Grisea, which is made from a diseased secretion of the intestine of a sperm whale.

But perhaps the best known of these is Oscilloccoccinum, which is the homeopathic "flu remedy" that is sold in all the health-food stores in those little white tubes. Oscilloccoccinum was actually discovered as a homeopathic remedy back in the mid 1930s, by the French physician Joseph Roy, who potentized the heart and liver of a Barbary Duck who was infected with the oscillococcus bacterium, thus the remedy's tongue-twisting name. In the past seventy years, the remedy has proven itself again and again to be a powerful tool helpful to those who are experiencing the onset of the symptoms of influenza.

Nosodes that come from disease tissues, whether those diseases are viral or bacterial, are very potent homeopathic medicines. They give us remedies like Tuberculinum, which is taken from bovine tissue that is infected with the mycobacterium tuberculosis. (It can also be created from the tubercular abscesses associated with the human tubercular bacillus. The two remedies, in proving by British homeopaths John Henry Clarke and James Compton Burnett, among others, showed little or no difference in their actions.)

Tuberculinum is a commonly used and very powerful nosode. Its action is said to especially affect the head, the mind, the lungs, the glands, and the larynx. This is a remedy commonly used for very sensitive patients, for those prone to respiratory ailments and failure to thrive. A deep fear of dogs is common in those needing this remedy. In modern homeopathy, it can often be given to children, especially to children with severe allergies.*

Another common nosode is Variolinum, which is made from smallpox. As the backache associated with the disease smallpox is considered to be especially severe, the remedy Variolinum is said to be helpful for those with pains in their back and legs.

Perhaps a more common use for this remedy is to combat what is called *vaccinosis*, or the ill effects of allopathic vaccinations.

There are many different nosodes among today's homeopathic remedies. Used correctly, they represent a unique and powerful section of the homeopathic pharmacy.

Sarcodes

Sarcodes are those homeopathic remedies that are taken from the healthy tissue of plants, animals, or humans. This would suggest a broad category containing the vast majority of homeopathic remedies. Strictly speaking, this may be true. Plant remedies that belong to this wide category include Guaiacum, which is made from gum resin of the lignum vitae, a tree native to the West Indies. The remedy Guaiacum is one of Hahnemann's own provings, and is considered to be a powerful anti-psoric remedy that is used commonly in cases involving gout and rheumatism.

---

* Today, some homeopaths are using the disease-based nosodes as constitutional remedies, giving the remedies in lower potencies and multiple doses. Other schools of thought hold that the nosodes are not constitutional remedies, but should more appropriately be used only in single doses, usually of a higher potency, such as a 1M. One thing is sure: a practitioner must avoid proving a nosode at all costs. These provings can be long lasting and very deep in their actions. Patients can be devastated by these provings. Therefore, I strongly believe that nosodes should not be used as constitutional treatments, but should be withheld until the need for them is clear. They may perhaps be more correctly considered to be our best treatments for those needing miasmic help. Nosodes will often break the chains of a miasm that have held a patient bound for many years. Since they work so well in single does, I cannot help but ask why they would be used in repeated low doses? It just seems crazy to me. And, as this practice is fairly new, we will not know its full ramifications until a generation passes and the children who today are being given Tuberculinum as if it were Phosphorus have grown and are showing the impact of their treatments. I would personally refuse treatment from any homeopath who felt that I was constitutionally a Tuberculinum or other disease-based nosode.

In that venoms and toxins taken from snakes and spiders are also considered to be "healthy" secretions, these remedies also belong to the category sarcode.

But the term sarcode is usually applied to specific remedies that are taken from animal organ tissue. Among these are the remedies Thyroidium, which is taken from a tincture made from the entire thyroid gland, and homeopathic Cortisone, which is potentized from the cortico-suprarenal hormone. The remedies taken from specific glands or secretions thereof can be somewhat narrow in their actions, seeking mostly to stimulate the gland from which it is taken.

Isodes

There are different sorts of remedies under the general category of *isode*. Some are useful homeopathic tools, while others stretch the boundaries of what may rightly be considered homeopathy.

The first subset of isopathic remedies is a very important little niche of homeopathic medicine in which known allergens are taken and potentized into homeopathic medicines. Today some homeopathic pharmaceutical firms carry a full range of these remedies, from cat hair, to dairy to different blends of pollens, which can be used to treat those who suffer from a specific allergy. In fact, some companies will actually make a remedy from the dander of your own pet, should you prove to be allergic to him, but love him too much to be willing to part.

This, it must be pointed out, does not represent a thorough understanding of what homeopathy is all about. While the basic premise seems to be clear enough—if you are allergic to a given substance, then it stands to reason that this same substance, if potentized, could remove your sensitivity to it—the process by which isopathic allergens are made ignores the fact that Hahnemann learned in first working with Sepia. Which is to say, until the remedy is made and clinically proven in its actions, we cannot be sure just what it will do. So when we take your dog's fur and potentize it, we cannot be sure that it will, in fact, have the action that we are hoping for. If the remedy were clinically proven, it might well show itself, like Sepia, to be a wonderful thing. But it might not.

In my experience, isopathic allergens do not work very well. They are fine if you are very allergic to cats and you have to visit your Aunt, who has ten of them. If you take the cat hair remedy before your visit, and, likely, often during your visit, the remedy will hold your allergies at bay for a time. But the remedy will not, unless you are very lucky and the general cat hair remedy is in a state of similarity with your own symptoms, remove the allergy from you.

Homeopathic allergens are sold in low potencies on the "X" scale of dilution. Taken with care in acute situations like that described above, they will do some good and little harm. Taken over time, they not only will fail to lift the allergy—as allergies can be one of the hardest forms of illness to treat—but they can prove themselves and actually increase the problem. Further, in that they are homeopathic remedies, when they are overused or used in combination, they carry the full implications of other misuses of homeopathic medicine.

One last note—if you are lactose intolerant and think that you can just take the dairy isode taken from milk or cheese and then eat what you want, you are in for a sad experience when you find that you cannot. Save yourself some discomfort and don't even try.

Another subset of isopathy has a name all its own: *tautopathy*. Tautopathic remedies are those taken from allopathic drugs, which themselves have already been given to the patient and caused some sort of harm. The idea, then, is the same as with the allergens listed above. It is thought that, if you give a remedy made from a potentized allopathic drug, then it will, in its action, reverse or remove the damage that has been caused by that drug. (Note that, while many of the proponents of tautopathy insist that it is not a form of isopathy, it really can't be considered as anything else, given the source material of the remedies, and the reasoning behind and methods of their use.)

Tautopathic remedies are fairly new to the homeopathic world. Many have been created since the 1960s. An example of a tautopathic remedy is Penicillinum, which is, of course, made from penicillin. This remedy is clinically associated with allergies, tubercular conditions and chronic fatigue syndrome, all of which themselves may be associated with the use of the drug penicillin.

Just as isopathic medicines can be made from allopathic drugs, they can be made from any other man-made toxic substance as well, including the wall-to-wall carpet in your house that constantly exudes toxic vapors. An example of just such a remedy is Naphthalinum, which is made from coal tar, which was, for many years, the basis of mothballs.

It may be said that all forms of isopathic medicine are somewhat suspect. This is most especially true of the final form of isopathic remedies, those known as *auto-isopathics*.

Now, again, at the first sound of it, this should make perfect homeopathic sense. After all, auto-isopathics are those remedies that are taken from the patient's own tissue, from his blood, hair, pus, spit, lymph, menstrual flow, semen, fingernails or toenails, or any other tissue taken from the body. What could, at first thought, seem a better use of the homeopathic principle than to take tissue from the patient, potentize it, and return it to the patient in the form of a medicine for all his ills?

The problem with this is that it does not represent true homeopathy. After all, the core principle by which homeopathy is practiced is "like cures like." In the use of homeopathic remedies, a remedy is found—from some other source—that has a life force that is in similarity to that of the patient. In isopathic remedies, we do not cure by the principle of "like cures like," but instead we insist that "the same cures the same." This, whether it works or not, is not homeopathy. It never can be.

A particular little cult has been built around what may be called "Urinum," which is the name given to any remedy made from a patient's own urine. While it is certainly true that the use of urine as a medicine is centuries old, it is also true that, as a homeopathic, it has never been proven to be of particular value.

The other problem with the use of isopathic medicines is that, once again, the medicine is merely potentized and then given to the patient with the assumption that it will do what is needed. But the remedy is not clinically proven first, so it is impossible to know what it will do, either in the patient's body or in anyone else's.

Who knows, isopathics may represent an exciting new system of medicine. But one thing is known—they are not homeopathics. They may be potentized like homeopathic medicines, but they are not clinically proven, repertorized, or given as homeopathics. And they never can be.

Options for Cure

The popularity that homeopathy has undergone in recent years has encouraged a great increase in the remedies available and in the many potencies in which remedies can be made. The result is that we have seen a dramatic increase of the remedies on the market, both the useful true homeopathics in the basic "X" and "C" scales of dilution, and odd new remedies in combination and isopathic forms.

Those who have studied or practiced homeopathy over a period of time will be well acquainted with the tried-and-true remedies, both the polycrests that are used so often that they, over time, seem to become members of the family, and the smaller remedies that are called into play as needed.

As you become more and more familiar with the remedies, and the archetypes implied by each, as you see the remedies in their actions in living, breathing beings, you will become more and more familiar with them in their full potential as well. In some cases, patients will always seem to respond well to the same small group of remedies, no matter the disease diagnosis. In other cases, a patient may need a wide range of remedies that seem to have no common context or action. And certainly, as our reach across the planet as a species increases, so will the source materials for new remedies.

While I have criticized the manner in which some new forms of remedies are made, I do not criticize those who explore the boundaries of homeopathy or the source materials for new homeopathic remedies.

With the remedies that we already have on hand in our full homeopathic pharmacy, it may honestly be said that there is no set of symptoms that homeopathic medicine cannot treat. It is, in its curative action, as wide and deep a system of medicine as allopathy is any day.

As students and practitioners alike further use and study the uses of the individual remedies, the practice of homeopathy can only become more effective. And, as the cannon of remedies is ever increased with the discovery of new sources for potentization, we can only have more options for cure.

CHAPTER SEVENTEEN

The Homeopath's Bookshelf

A generation ago, it was very difficult to find any books on the subject of home-opathy. After you bought the two or three that you found at your health-food store, you would have to scour the shelves of used books stores and antique stores (a surprisingly good source, since many of the books on homeopathy had been published a hundred years ago) in order to find anything on the subject. And when you did find a book, you bought it, no questions asked. Over the years I collected books on the homeopathic treatment of horses, and learning to dose homeopathically based on the phases of the moon. Neither was of much practical use to me, but back in those days before eBay, you pretty much had to be happy with whatever you could find.

Today, the problem has reversed itself. Every publishing company, large or small, wants at least one book on the subject for their backlist. So, while homeopathy remains a niche area in publishing, there are now literally hundreds of titles available. Add to this the fact that old books never die anymore, but simply go on to live on the Internet, and you have an enormous wealth of information available.

So the problem now becomes what to choose? Which books are best? Which books belong on the bookshelf of every person interested in homeopathy?*

As with anything else homeopathic, there is no easy general answer here. The books needed by a particular reader, of course, depend upon the goals of that reader. Those who want to know enough about homeopathy to be of some use to themselves and their family have one set of needs. Those who want to practice homeopathy professionally have another set altogether.

But both groups begin at the same place.

---

* Please turn to the Resource Guide at the end of the book for a complete listing of the books discussed here, along with information on homeopathic organizations, websites and suppliers of homeopathic goods.

The *Organon*

The first book on the subject of homeopathy that everyone should read is the *Organon of Medicine* by Dr. Samuel Hahnemann. And, for me, there is only one edition of this book that anyone needs to own, and everyone needs to own it. It is the relatively new translation of the German text that was edited by Wenda Brewster O'Reilly. It was not until this book, precisely entitled the *Organon of the Medical Art*, was published back in 1996 that Americans had a good translation (by Steven Decker) of the original text. But with this edition, there is at last a publication of Hahnemann's greatest work that is easy to read and easy to understand.*

As British homeopath Jeremy Sherr writes in the foreword, "Organon contains the word 'or,' which in Hebrew means 'light.' In the beginning God made light which, endowed with love and truth, fertilized life with the seeds of source. In the medical world, Hahnemann's *Organon* represents this light. Here lies the organic origin, the creative core of true healing. . . . Universal law forms the basis of homeopathy. Becoming a homeopath does not depend on the study of materia medica. It is not defined by prescribing potentized remedies, nor is it reliant on remembering the repertory. It is the living and understanding of these laws which endows our medical practice."

> "It is recommended . . . that the *Organon* be read twice a year for the first fifty years of practice, and thenceforth once a year."

Later in his foreword, Sherr notes, "It is recommended by the old homeopaths that the *Organon* be read twice a year for the first fifty years of practice, and thenceforth once a year."

Those who are students of homeopathy should read it even more often. The *Organon of Medicine* contains everything that Hahnemann has to say, both on the subject of medicine and on homeopathy.

When I first heard about the book, I thought that it would be an encyclopedia. I ordered it, and, when it arrived, it turned out to be a very slim volume. Even this new edition, with very eye-easy print and an excellent index (for which I am always grateful), still comes in at just about four hundred pages.

The thing that can be confusing about the *Organon* is that there's more than one of them. By this I don't mean that there's an *Organon of Cooking* and an *Organon of*

---

* It is not my intent to do commercials in these pages, and this is the only specific edition of any type of book that I ever recommend. This new translation, however, stands head and shoulders above any that have heretofore available in English. Further, the book has been edited and structured in such a way as to enhance understanding and readability. *One last thing, remember that some of the best things that Hahnemann has to say he says in his footnotes.* Don't skip them. Footnotes are good things.

Gardening, I mean that, instead of writing multiple books over the course of his career, Hahnemann instead went back and re-edited and added to the same book over and over again. There are, altogether, six editions of the *Organon*. Those wanting to read the complete homeopathic philosophy as Hahnemann shaped it over the years will want to either own the sixth edition, or a volume that combines the fifth and sixth editions.

I do want to warn you going in that, even with the new translation, the *Organon* can be a tough go. It remains couched in the language of two hundred years ago. Perhaps what is needed is a paraphrase edition to sit along side the translations, sort of a "Good News for Modern Homeopaths."

Some homeopathic educators tend to think that new students should not begin with Hahnemann's work because of its difficulty. I disagree. Too many students start with home guides and never get past them. They learn a simplified version of homeopathic philosophy that never quite serves them as it should. Worse, when health crises come—and they will—those who never learned homeopathic philosophy are left flipping from page to page in their home guides, hoping to get lucky with a remedy.

As Jeremy Sherr wrote, "It is the living and the understanding of the (universal) laws which endows our medical practice." That holds true for "professional" and lay homeopaths alike.

The Materia Medica

It is important that you approach a Materia Medica with the right frame of mind. No Materia Medica is what the *Organon* is—a statement of core principles and universal laws. Instead, each Materia Medica represents the notes that a specific homeopath has taken over a lifetime of using the remedies.*

To refer to any specific Materia Medica—and there are many out there—is like calling that practitioner on the phone and asking him questions about individual remedies. Each Materia Medica lists the remedies in alphabetical order. Within each listing is first an overview of the remedy and its actions. This is followed by a more detailed breakdown that travels from the top of the patient's head down to the bottom of his feet, listing the specific symptoms associated with the action of the remedy to every part of the body affected by that remedy. At the end of the listing, you will find further information about that remedy. In some Materia Medicas, you will find infor-

---

* The concept of a Materia Medica, with its listings of the full uses for different medicines, is not original to homeopathy. Herbal practitioners were writing Materia Medicas in ancient Rome. Hahnemann borrowed the concept and structure of these works in creating his own Materia Medica of homeopathic remedies.

mation on specific cases for which the practitioner made use of the remedy. In most you will find information on the effectiveness of one potency versus another, the approximate period of time for which each dose is effective and how the particular remedy works when used before or after another remedy—what remedies antidote its action, and what remedies help complete the case.

In other words, Materia Medicas are very valuable things. But remember that each is simply the informed opinion of one practitioner. This means several things. First, I strongly suggest that you should have on hand more than one Materia Medica, so that you can compare and contrast the information from two or more. In fact, I suggest that you collect as many different Materia Medicas as you can afford. You cannot have too many of them. Each has its unique advice to give, each will reveal some different aspect of a remedy that may be very valuable to you. In that you will only need one edition of the *Organon* for your whole lifetime (that's why I think you should just buy it in hardback to begin with), you should have as many different Materia Medicas as you can.

Second, as you learn more and more about homeopathy, you will no doubt find a Materia Medica written by a person who thinks more or less as you do. Hang on to that one and refer to it often.

Third, in today's world, we have begun to see the publication of a new form of Materia Medicas, ones that are sources of secondary information. By this I mean that, instead of being the original work for a specific practitioner, they are the product of clever editors, who combine the information contained within several old Materia Medicas into something "new." This is not to say that these books are not valuable in their way, simply that, in my opinion, something of the practitioner's passion is lost in the translation.

Finally, on the subject of Materia Medicas, I am sad to say that James Tyler Kent never wrote a Materia Medica. It would have had a prominent place on my bookshelf. Luckily, he did teach Materia Medica to his students and his class notes have been published in a volume called *Lectures on Homeopathic Materia Medica*. That is a reference work well worth owning. You will refer to it again and again.

Repertory

A Repertory is a very important tool in homeopathic case management. The information contained within a Repertory interlocks with that in the Materia Medica, giving you all the information you need, in theory at least, to select an appropriate remedy and use it correctly.

The Repertory is something like a dictionary of symptoms. Any symptom, for something as general as a headache to something as specific as a cough that occurs only from three until four o'clock in the afternoon will be listed in the pages of this book. Next to the symptom will be listed the names of all the remedies that have the ability to create that symptom in a proving. And the remedies are graded in their importance to that symptom as well, which is to say by how powerfully they have the ability to impact that symptom.

Like a Materia Medica, a Repertory is the product of one practitioner and his life-time of experience in using homeopathic remedies. Because they are the product of one practitioner, they can differ greatly, both in the way they are structured and in the information contained within.*

Some are structured so that the symptoms are listed from the top of the head downward, like the listings in the Materia Medica. Others, like dictionaries, list the symptoms in alphabetical order. I personally prefer the alphabetical order.

The thing to remember about Repertories is that, as the product of an individual mind that was committed to print years ago, they are not going to bend to your needs, to work with a Repertory, you are going to have to take it on its own terms. In other words, if that particular Repertory separates the impact that particular foods have in the patient's body (under "stomach") from the particular foods that the patient craves (under "mind"), then you are just going to have to remember where each is located.

Even more than with a Materia Medica—since all Materia Medicas are struc-tured in similar fashion—when you choose your Repertory, you are going to have to choose one that was created by someone who thinks as you do, who would put his socks in the same drawer that you would. If you can find that Repertory, then you will have a much easier time using it and locating the individual symptoms that you need. Remember, you can take the best case in the world, but if you can't locate the rubrics (those are the individual listings) in the Repertory that will help you choose a remedy, then you're not going to do much good, are you?

I believe that you will only need one good Repertory. And that, once you find it, you should do the very best job that you can to become just as familiar with it as you possibly can. When you get it, practice with it. Pretend that someone has a headache, and just look through the many, many rubrics that pertain to headache. Get familiar so that, when you are under pressure, when someone is in crisis, you can research the case quickly and well. If you can learn your way around one Repertory—really get to know it—you will be able to do a great deal more than can those who own a dozen and can't make sense out of any of them.

---

* The creation of the Repertory is credited both to Clemens Maria Franz von Boenninghausen and to Georg Heinrich Gottlieb Jahr. Both published a Repertory in the early 1830s. Each worked independently of the other. And the two Repertories approached the structuring of the symptoms in a different way. Jahr's Repertory presented the symptoms in the manner in which is more or less still in use today. Most famously, it was, in structure, the basis for Kent's own.

And those who never get to know a Repertory, who wait for a crisis to try and learn homeopathy—they end up reaching for one of those damned home guides.

Those Damned Home Guides

First, let me swear that I really have nothing against homeopathic home guides.* I have written two myself and I think that they are both pretty good.

You just have to make sure that, as your refer to them, you don't try to make them be something more than they are. These are very simplistic books. They are written in order to help beginning students learn how to deal with very simple ailments. They do so by reducing the actions of a given remedy down to one or two sentences, and by listing only maybe six remedies of a given condition. Now, in reality, a Materia Medica will list page after page about each remedy, and a Repertory may list fifty or more remedies for a given symptom, but the home guide lives in a world in which all can be set right if you simply have a home kit of thirty remedies, all in the same potency.

> The other real issue I have with home guides is that no one ever reads them.

Sometimes it works, sometimes it doesn't.

The other real issue I have with home guides is that no one ever reads them. As I said, I've written two of them, and I can't say that I have ever met anyone who has taken the time to read all the information contained in the first section of either book. Instead they read the second section—the part that lists the most common remedies for common illness (something I refer to as using as "homeopathic Band-Aid")—and they only read that during moments of crisis. Little Johnny has the croup at two in the morning and *now* the parents develop an interest in homeopathy. It's no wonder that homeopathic home guides are of so little value, in that they are not even used to their limited potential.

So you can have as few or as many as you want. But you must actually read the ones you own. And use them with an air of caution. Where Repertories and Materia Medicas will contain some similar and some different information from volume to volume, home guides may have absolutely nothing in common at all. Some offer the most alarming information as to what they consider "homeopathy" to be. Others, in their limited listings for individual ailments, will not have a single remedy in common from listing to listing. Many read as if they, like the *Organon*, were translated from other languages, and that they are still awaiting their definitive English translation.

---

* I actually collect antique home guides. I love them. I love the names they give their ailments and, especially, the special diets for "dropsy," etc.

Other Books

If you have a copy of the *Organon*, a few Materia Medicas, and a really good Repertory, then you are pretty well fixed. However, there are some other books that will be of help to you and that belong on your homeopathic bookshelf.

The first of these is *A Dictionary of Homeopathic Medical Terminology* by Jay Yasgur. This excellent little book will define some of the more exotic terms that you will find in the Repertory and Materia Medica, such exciting things as "barber's itch," "erythrism," and "omphalitis" (which is a lovely word for an inflammation of the navel) will be fully explained in its pages. If you prefer, another way to go is to get an old medical dictionary at a book sale. You can usually buy one very cheap. The fact that it uses antiquated medical terms will make it of little value to an allopath, but of great help to you. In fact, the older the dictionary, the better.

Books on homeopathic theory can certainly be very helpful, although none of them approaches the *Organon* in fully exploring and explaining homeopathy. However, there is much to be learned in the books of George Vithoulkas, Edward Whitmont, and Margery Blackie, among others. Again, with the many volumes now available, I think that it is best if you just thumb through them and choose the ones you like. You can never read too many books on homeopathy if you keep in mind that the last word in homeopathy is Hahnemann's and that those who claim to have something totally new to add are wrong. Hahnemann wrote the best possible book on homeopathy, the rest of us are just rewriting it over and over again, adding our little bits of insight.

Take a look at the Resource Guide at the end of this book for more information on the books and authors mentioned here.

Computer Software

I put computer software into the same category as home guides.* Software that contains every Materia Medica and Repertory ever known can be a wonderful tool. Trouble is that, in my experience, this tool is not being used by skilled homeopaths who have spent years and years repertorizing by hand, turning the pages of the book and writing out the rubrics, no, they tend to be used by people who never bothered to learn how to solve a case on their own, because they learned early on that they could get the computer to do the work for them. This makes them like big, huge, really, really detailed home guides, but the principle remains the same: if you don't understand homeopathy, if you don't live it, then no computer is going to make up for that fact.

---

* What it comes down to is shortcuts. When it comes to homeopathy, I don't like shortcuts.

Doing the work yourself, getting out your books and piling them around you as you write your notes on a legal pad is good for you. Work and work until you are satisfied that you have done a good job and found the right remedy. It builds your mind and, over time, makes you more and more knowledgeable. There is no way that your computer can teach you homeopathy by flashing the information for you. Maybe if I'd ever found a type of software that was organized well or excited me in any way I'd use it. But I'm still working at my kitchen table.

CHAPTER EIGHTEEN

Taming the Beast

If you have made the decision to become more involved with homeopathy, then there is only one real hurdle that remains, well, two really. The first has to do with the fact that, in all reality, you are going to have to find yourself some sort of homeopath to depend upon in times of need. And the second is that, at some point and to some extent, you are going to have to deal with the homeopathic community.

Stalking the Homeopath

The more important of these two issues concerns finding the right homeopath for your needs.

This is never easy, and it can be made a whole lot more difficult if you happen to find yourself living in any of these United States that lack ocean views.

You see, in our country, while control of medicine is left up to the federal government, the definition of and control over the practice of different forms of medicine is left up to the states. So while homeopathic remedies are legally considered over-the-counter medication in all fifty states, it has been left up to the states to control who can practice the form of medicine that relies on these remedies. Now this, of course, doesn't make much sense, since it creates an environment in many states in which anyone can walk into a health-food store and buy nearly any remedy they want and take it as they please, no matter what potential harm they may cause themselves, but they may not be able to work with professionals who could oversee the safety and efficacy of the treatment. And in the states in which homeopathy is a gray area in the law, in which it hasn't yet been dealt with adequately, you will find that it is often the case that those who know the most about homeopathy cannot legally practice it, even if they have some sort of medical degree, like a nursing degree or a naturopath's certification, while those who *are* practicing it are the kooks and quacks who will be happy to practice without a license—the very ones that the state *should* be preventing from practicing.

So it can be a very difficult thing to find a skilled homeopath, most especially if you want to be able to receive insurance co-payments for your treatments. Which is an issue of greater and greater importance as the cost of a visit to a homeopath continues to skyrocket.

To my best knowledge—and I may be wrong about this, as laws in individual states may have changed—it is legal for medical doctors (M.D.s) to include homeopathic remedies as a part of their practice in all fifty states. The problem here is that it is sometimes the case that the doctors using the remedies have very little actual training in their use. There is not, for instance, any test that they have to pass to prove proficiency. No, it is felt that their license to practice allopathic medicine surely gives them the knowledge needed to handle the remedies safely and effectively. Even though the remedies in question work in a manner opposite to the medicines that the doctor was trained to use. And even though homeopathy is a complex field of study that was likely not even mentioned in medical school. So you will find the occasional doctor who has taken a few classes and decides to call himself a homeopath, even though his knowledge of homeopathy is weak at best.

In some states, naturopaths are allowed to practice homeopathy. And sometimes that works out well, since naturopaths are taught at least a basic understanding of homeopathy as part of their training.

But often naturopaths grow confused by the sheer sweep of their studies. You see, where medical doctors tend to narrow their field of work down to one organ or system in the body, naturopaths study natural medicine as a whole, with nutrition, herbal medicine, homeopathy, energy medicine, and other fields of study all included. It is for this reason that this field of study was once called "Eclectic Medicine." So it should come as no surprise when I say that my problem with naturopaths is that they all too often try to be all things to all people. I have known many who mixed homeopathic remedies with herbal treatments (which are always, by their very nature, allopathic) on a daily basis. And most especially when faced with a health crisis, they tend to throw everything including the homeopathic kitchen sink at the problem, often so muddling the case as to make it nearly incurable.

I knew one excellent homeopath who had moved to our country from a foreign land. She came from a family of homeopaths and had studied all her life to become quite an impressive practitioner. For a while, she practiced homeopathy in sort of a black-market fashion, from a little room that required all but a secret knock in order to gain entry. Finally, the stress of practicing medicine in our country without a license wore her down and she went off to the Pacific Northwest to get her naturopathic degree. When she returned and set up shop, I discovered to my great sorrow and dismay that this excellent classical homeopath had been morphed into a mediocre naturopath.

Honestly, it is very difficult for any student to withstand the studies required in order to become either an allopathic medical doctor or a naturopath and still, at the end of those studies, be able to practice homeopathy as Hahnemann practiced it.

> It is very difficult for any student to withstand the studies required in order to become either a medical doctor or a naturopath and still, at the end of those studies, be able to practice homeopathy as Hahnemann practiced it.

There is something to the fact that those who became homeopaths early on were rebelling, openly and actively rebelling and spitting on the ground as they did so, against what they disdainfully called the "old school" of medicine, allopathy, that gave their practice of the new art of homeopathy such power. It was power born of radical ideas, new discoveries, and pure rage.

Today, many of those galumphing their way out of naturopathic schools seem lacking in this sort of passion. Indeed, they seem, for the most part, rather passive, motivated by a vague notion of "doing good." They lack the specific training in classical homeopathy that they need to fulfill that intention, however. The very fact that here in the United States we have no legal designation of "homeopath" and no school that can both train and certify homeopaths leaves us forever dependant upon those who, with some other sort of medical training and degree, manage to some degree or other to incorporate homeopathy into their practice.

All of this, of course, makes the search for a good homeopathic practitioner all the more difficult.

But there are good homeopaths out there, good practitioners to be found with every sort of medical background. But you are going to have to find them for yourself. (The Resource Guide at the end of this book should be of some help to you in listing organizations, such as the National Center for Homeopathy, which makes lists of homeopathic practitioners available.)

In my opinion, the first thing to do is to try and find out who in your state can legally practice homeopathy. This, in and of itself, is not always an easy thing to find out. I would start by calling some sort of holistic medical practice. They almost always know the lay of the land. It can be valuable to call the state capital as well, as they will be able to supply you with the actual law.

Then you need to contact your insurance company and find out whether or not they cover homeopathy. If they do not, demand to know why not and demand that they begin to cover it immediately. This likely won't do you much good, if you are the only one making this demand, but if enough voices join your own a change may one day be made.

At this point, you will know what kind or kinds of practitioner you can choose from in your state and whether or not the cost of the visit will be out of your own pocket.

From here, you have to contact some offices and ask a lot of questions. If they— the receptionist or whoever is thrown between you and the doctor—is unwilling or unable to answer your questions and someone else is not quickly found who can, move on. You will want to know what kind of homeopathy they practice. If they, as they usually do, say "classical homeopathy," ask what that means and listen carefully to their answer. If it isn't a good one, move on. Find out how long the first session will last, how it will be run, and how long it will take from there for you to get some form of diagnosis and remedy. Make sure that you are satisfied with the information you are given. Find out the cost of the first session and ask if the doctor uses homeopathic software, or if they repertorize the old-fashioned way. The old-fashioned way is better, but I have nothing against the use of software, as long as the treatment is not completely based on the information it yields.

And go by your gut. Does this office seem to be genuinely concerned with your well-being, or is money being mentioned too often or too soon? Do you want to trust your health or the health of your child to the people in this office? Only you can know the answer to these questions.

The Care and Feeding of Your Homeopath

At some point, you are going to just have to bite the bullet and go to see a practitioner.

And remember as you go that there are many different ways to practice homeopathy. There are the "classical" homeopaths who will adhere strictly to the Three Laws of Cure that we've already discussed. And there are many others who practice something that they call homeopathy, but may or may not be based on the Three Laws. The country is filled with practitioners who will use crystals and pendulums to help them select your remedy. Beware of them.

I believe that the more classically trained a homeopath is—no matter how they received that classical education—the better homeopath he or she will be. Adherence to the Three Laws does not make a homeopath narrower in his practice or less able to deal with the health challenges of today's world—and these are two arguments you will hear again and again from those who do not follow the laws and who wish to rail against Hahnemann's practice of homeopathy—rather, it frees them to work cleanly and safely in restoring a patient to health, which is the whole goal of homeopathy.

Even within the realm of what is considered "classical" homeopathy, there are different philosophies of practice. Some practitioners will use single doses or wait a very long time between doses of a remedy. Others may give the remedy more often at first and wait to see a reaction on the part of the patient before tapering off the remedy's use. Still others will use only high potencies, and others will use only low. There are practitioners who will stress the use of the so-called LM potencies—specially pre-pared remedies in liquid form that are taken daily for a month or longer at a time. LM potencies are said to be even safer and gentler in their action than are the traditional remedies and they are often used in cases involving increased sensitivity on the part of a patient or great depletion.

All of these paths can be pathways to cure. As long as your homeopath has been well trained, his or her own clinical experience with the remedies will guide that homeopath in the selection and use of remedies. All the different variations of these "classical" methods of treatment will work, and, in the hands of a trained and capable homeopath, can lead to a cure that is rapid, gentle, and permanent.

From here we move on to groups of practitioners for whom the same conclusion cannot be drawn. These are the practitioners that Hahnemann himself would have called "half-homeopaths." These are those who use homeopathic remedies, but whose use of them falls outside the Three Laws. They fall into three different categories of "half-homeopaths."

The first group is perhaps most common. They are the "allopathic homeopaths."

These practitioners have lost sight of the fact that, in homeopathic medicine, we are always to treat the patient, and never treat the disease. These practitioners will make a great show of using the latest technology in all its forms, turning to every med-ical test available and every bit of software that they can find. Now, in and of itself, this use of technology is not a bad thing. I am all for technology that can enhance our abilities, whether it be in medicine or any other field. However, when technology replaces appropriate training and necessary work, when it ceases to be a tool and becomes the single avenue of thought or insight, then trouble begins.

These are the practitioners who will not give you a drug diagnosis, as the more classical homeopaths will. Instead, you will get a disease diagnosis from them and, like allopaths, they will then use the name of the disease as a method by which they map your experience of your illness. Instead of considering the entire homeopathic phar-macy as potential tools to your cure, they will only consider those remedies that are said to work for this particular disease. So what guides and controls them in their work to bring about a much needed cure in your life are not the specifics of your case and how the symptoms have come upon you and changed your life, no, what guides them will be a single word—the name of that disease itself. And, if they have the diagnosis wrong? If they are using the wrong word to describe you in your diseased state? Then they will likely be considering the wrong remedies and no cure can possibly result. It's just that simple.

A real warning to you that you are dealing with an allopath wearing a home-opath's white coat will be when the practitioner talks a good deal about your disease and calls it by name. Says things like, "Yes, I have seen other cases of irritable bowel syndrome and Sulphur has always been a good choice." That tells you, in the first place, he is thinking of you as a case of irritable bowel syndrome, which is not a good thing. And that he is narrowing down his choice of remedies not based on your collective symptoms and their similarity to Sulphur's actions, but based upon past experience of this *disease*. This is someone who may be an excellent doctor, but who is not a good homeopath. Walk away.

The second group, the polypharmacists, have forgotten that they should not give more than one remedy at a time. That they will not be able to tell which remedy has brought about what action if they give multiple remedies.

If you are in one of their offices and you object to the idea of taking multiple remedies simultaneously, you will find that these practitioners have heard that argument before. And they have their answers ready. They will say that, in our polluted world, our bodies face so many more stresses so we need to take more than one remedy at a time to combat them.

Don't fall for this reasoning. It is completely inane. Are we to believe that they have somehow developed the ability to know the unknowable? First, in practicing what they call homeopathy through the use of multiple remedies, they infer that they can somehow tell that their patient will need more than one remedy before they have given them *any*. Second, they seem to have somehow developed the ability to be able to unravel the impact of polypharmacy and know the actions of each remedy used so that they can track those actions toward a cure. This is just simply not possible.

Also, the idea that we are sicker or less sick than humans were a century or a millennia ago is also just unknowable. And in all actuality it is also irrelevant. The practitioner is to deal with the patient in front of him and to restore him to health. It is that simple. Whether or not people in Germany two hundred years ago, those treated by Hahnemann, were healthier or not in general because of the cleanliness of their environment could not be less an issue in deciding how we proceed with this patient. Whether or not pollution is playing an active or passive role in this patient's health may or may not be an issue, as his system may be quite strong enough to overcome the challenge of pollution. This is part of what the qualified homeopath must discover as he takes the patient's case and then considers it through repertorization.

To be brief, polypharmacy is never a good idea. It never works. It will never work. Avoid it and those who practice it.

Now the third group, those who practice by prescribing a set number of doses of a given remedy over a set number of days, these practitioners really get my goat. Let's call them the "overdosers."

Remember, more cases are spoiled—which is a nice term really, but by "spoiled" I mean that a patient who could have been cured is not cured and continues to suffer—by a practitioner not knowing when to stop giving a remedy than by any other method.

So here we have another group of practitioners who is claiming to know the unknowable. This time they are telling us to believe that they are able to predict just how much medicine will be needed to do the job.

Nonsense.

There is no way to know this. You have to give the remedy, and then wait and watch. How long you wait and watch depends upon two things: how serious the condition is right now and whether or not you can afford to wait for very long and what sort of remedy you have given, and how swift or slow its action is known to be.

All remedies should be taken *as needed.* That means that the action of the remedy and the reaction of the patient need to be observed and noted. That means that the practitioner does not get to sell you a vial of medicine and then tell you to take it twice a day for a month and then come back for a follow-up. Now, in acute cases, it is sometimes just easier to say, "Take this three times a day until you feel better, then call me." Even that's just sloppy, if you ask me, but it really isn't that awful. But in chronic cases requiring constitutional care, it is really in my opinion just unbelievably shoddy for a so-called homeopath to push the patient out the door clutching a medicine that may well work in just a dose or two and then spend twenty-eight days more repeating that dose into an aggravation, a proving, and the possible spoiling of the case. These practitioners turn many people off to homeopathy through their limp understanding of its practice. And that's actually the best possible outcome. Worse, they can come upon a patient who just keeps trusting them and just takes the remedy as directed and becomes very sick as a result.

Notice that each of the three groups I have outlined above have elected to ignore one Law of Cure. The first group, the allopathic homeopaths, ignores Similar, and gives a remedy not based on the patient's symptoms, but based upon their disease. This does not work. The second group of half-homeopaths, the polypharmacists, ignores Simplex, and gives more than one remedy at a time. A variation on this is the practitioner who gives one homeopathic remedy at a time, but couples it with herbal remedies or allopathic medicines. Polypharmacy still results. This does not work either. The final group, the overdosers, ignores Minimum and gives a remedy until they, the practitioner, are ready to stop and not until the needs of the patient have been fulfilled. This does not work.

Even worse are those practitioners who break more than one Law. Who will give multiple medicines on a rigid schedule not based on need. Or who give a mix of medicines based upon a disease diagnosis. As a practitioner breaks another Law of Cure, they are taking another step away from homeopathy, until they are not even "half-homeopaths" but can in no way claim to be homeopaths at all. These folks are just plain dangerous. I hope you will avoid them.

Homeopathic Veterinarians—A Special Horror

To my knowledge, there is no worse single group of homeopaths, quasi-homeopaths, and faux-homeopaths than the homeopathic vets. My only advice, based on my past willingness to work with several of them, is to run. Run far and run fast and do not let your beloved pet get into their clutches.

Now I want to believe that somewhere in this world there are many skilled and loving homeopathic vets who have nothing but the highest quality of care to offer. And I have looked high and low for these practitioners, but in fifteen years of searching, I have yet to find one.

I have yet to find a homeopathic vet who really knows and loves the practice of homeopathy. And who passionately loves animals as well. Instead, I have found them to be an overpriced lot who sit at their computers entering symptoms and waiting for the machine to tell them what to do. Many also have learned a new trick of selling the remedies direct to their customers. Those customers who buy these remedies will find that they have been charged twice as much for a few pellets of remedy in a glass tube than they would have paid for a full tube at the health-food store.

Honestly, I would love to be proven wrong in my opinion of these people. And I still live in hope, as my dog Django is my pride and joy. But until my own experience changes, it is my strong advice that if you are going to use homeopathy as a primary form of treatment for your animals, then I *strongly* suggest that you learn enough homeopathy if not to just treat them yourself, then to at least know when you are being given bad advice.

Remember, the great trick to treating animals is being able to communicate with a being who cannot simply tell you what is wrong. Perhaps this is what makes the homeopathic vet's job so seemingly impossible. But you know your animal better than anyone else. Over the years of living with an animal, an almost telepathic bond is formed. Trust that bond. And trust yourself as you learn homeopathy that you can learn to support your animal's health homeopathically, even if you must, from time to time, call upon the help of an allopathic or homeopathic vet.

> The only real mistake, no matter which school of medicine you ultimately advocate, is waiting for the health crisis to get involved, get educated. That only makes the process much harder, and much more likely to fail.

It is just the same as treating your children or anyone else you love. You are going to have to be the responsible party here. That means learning it yourself. Selecting the remedy yourself if you have to, or at least overseeing the selection and use of the remedy.

And, truthfully, whether you go the homeopathic route for yourself, your children and your pets, or you stay with the allopathic medicine that you already know, if you are going to navigate the savage waters of our health system, you are going to have to be an advocate, a rabble-rouser and, likely, a practitioner anyway, so you might as well get started. The only real mistake, no matter which school of medicine you ultimately advocate, is waiting for the health crisis to get involved, get educated. That only makes the process much harder, and much more likely to fail.

The Essence of the Homeopath

I don't want to leave you with the impression that I have no respect for anyone who practices homeopathy. This is simply not the case. There is no one that I respect more than the working homeopath, whether they are a lay practitioner—and some of the finest homeopaths I have ever known were lay practitioners who knew much more about homeopathy than the medical professionals around them—or a nurse practitioner, a doctor, a chiropractor, or a naturopath. It has been my experience that the type of medical degree, or, even, the existence of a medical degree, tells you nothing about the skill and knowledge and dedication of a given practitioner. What will often tell you the most is their heart. Their willingness to not always be right, if it means that their patient can be made well. Their willingness to stick with a case, repertorize it again, consider it again and again, until the patient is made well. The number of times that the practitioner makes himself or herself available to the patient in person or by phone. And the importance that the practitioner places on money, most especially on acquiring it.

There is a story I like to tell, which, to me, defines the essence of a homeopath.

It takes place more than twenty years ago in Edinburgh, Scotland.

I had traveled to Scotland with a friend and we were together attending the annual Fringe Festival. Now, a week or so before, we had been in London and had had dinner with friends on a houseboat on the Thames. And I had afterward come down with a terrible cold. As we drove from London to Edinburgh, I sneezed and sneezed and sneezed. As a result of a particularly bad sneeze, I threw my back out. So, instead of attending the Fringe Festival, I laid on the floor of our hotel room, moaning and watching the Tour de France on one of three television stations available.

I did the best I could throughout Saturday trying to get over the cold and, especially, the back pain. When my friend returned to our room from some opera or theater performance, I made her hurl the mattress from my bed down on the floor so that I could have a more comfortable surface on which to suffer.

By Sunday morning, I knew that I couldn't take it anymore. I needed help. There I was in a foreign land without my remedies, without my books, and I was in pain. I decided to try the phone book.

I looked under "Homeopaths" and found several listed. Luckily, the very first one I called answered the phone. I told her my problem and where I was located and she told me that she had her office nearby. Even though it was Sunday morning, she agreed to go and open her office and to meet us there. We drove over and found a beautiful old stone building with a hand-painted wooden sign over the storefront that read "Homeopath."

The Scottish homeopath, I have long since forgotten her name, took the case clearly and quickly—after all, it was a simple acute situation—and gave me the remedy that very quickly put me back on my feet and allowed me, two days later, to get on my jet and fly back home.

Now, that's a homeopath.

She worked when she was needed, without fuss, she charged a fair rate for her skill, but there were no intake forms or special fees for the first visit. She put the vial of pellets in my hand and told me how to take them. And, in short order, without undue fuss, she put things right.

Over the years, I have met many such practitioners. I know that they do exist. I hope that you can find one for yourself and for your family, because such practitioners are full partners with their patients in attaining and maintaining optimal health.

The Homeopathic Community

Let me say from the first that I do not believe that I have met so many truly fine people in any group related to any particular belief or creed as I have in the homeopathic community. This is particularly true of the laypeople who are the backbone of this community.

After all, these are the patients who fill the practitioners' offices, these are the students who fill the classrooms, and these are likely the readers of books like this one. The vast majority of the students that I have met have been driven toward homeopathy by some failing in our nation's health-care system. Many have personally experienced the failure of allopathic treatments or have been deemed, for one reason or another, to be untreatable and therefore have no choice but to try alternative treatments. Others lack health insurance, and therefore lack access to the health-care system and have to use methods by which they can self-treat, in the hope of maintaining their good health. Therefore they come to homeopathy for very good reasons. And they very often find in homeopathy the solution to their health issues.

This gives these people a certain zeal for homeopathy, and a vast patience for those who come into homeopathy after them. They will help by freely giving whatever information is asked of them, whatever support is needed.

This aspect of our nation's homeopathic community is both welcoming and healthy.

The breakdown comes further up the chain. It has to do with those medical professionals who may or may not actually practice homeopathy, but who are part of the community. And with those who actually run the national and regional groups, those who—like so many, especially in niche communities, get a little of what they perceive as power and just plain don't know how to handle it—all too often see it as their job to grant or deny access to the information on homeopathy that their particular organization has to offer.

Homeopathic Organizations

Just look at a map of the homeopathic organizations in our nation and you are looking at a map of the Middle Ages. Fiefdoms everywhere. Each ruled over by a particular Duke or Duchess, King or Queen. And in the mix are several Popes or pretenders to the throne, all of whom consider themselves to be infallible.

It is a painful thing to watch how these organizations treat each other, and to hear the awful gossip and rumors that flow from group to group. In the eyes of many of these Medieval organizations, the single worst thing another group can do is be successful. That they simply cannot abide. Instead of modeling themselves after allopathic organizations, which have so successfully closed ranks on many occasions for the overall good of allopathic medicine, homeopathic organizations simply don't seem capable of getting past their own self-interest.

In the short term, this may be good for a single group, but in the long term it is just terrible for homeopathy.

It can be painful to watch how these same national and regional organizations treat the lay homeopaths. How a layperson who has studied homeopathy for half their lifetime can be told that they may not speak from the same podium with someone who went to a questionable college is quite beyond me. I have seen laypeople rudely interrupted, corrected, censored and, if they will not sit in the back of the homeopathic bus, simply asked to leave. I have seen laypeople who had the skill and intelligence to teach a particular class be refused *admission* to that class because it was just for medical professionals. And I will not support this sort of thing. Not with my membership, or my money.

Both are important issues here. On the one hand, these organizations want your money—they cannot exist without it—but on the other hand, they want you to sit down and shut up and be thankful that they will let you pay to attend their beginner class again and again. All passionate students of homeopathy deserve something better.

It is my belief that homeopathic organizations have to *deserve* to exist, like any other organization. The fact that they exist at all is not reason enough to support them and to enable their actions with our money. As we deserve excellence in our practitioners, we also deserve it from our own organizations, our own community. And often we don't get it, particularly from the larger, more deeply entrenched of these organizations. Often, when criticized, the most heavy-handed organizations are the very first to run for cover behind the fact that they are largely volunteer run (forget the fact that these "volunteers" are the very physicians and pharmacy owners whose skills and products are advertised in that organization's booklet, and are therefore filling their offices and selling their remedies based upon the fact that they volunteer a few hours a year to the organization), and therefore we have no right to expect anything much from them.

So these organizations, which call themselves "professional" when it suits them and "volunteer run" when they need to lower expectations on the part of their membership and the public, pretty much end up failing the very community they supposedly exist to support. Too often, their sole goal becomes the continued survival of their own organization. Too often, instead of meeting the needs of their own membership and of the larger homeopathic community, they meet only their own.

Grassroots Groups

The smaller grass-root organizations tend to be much better and more responsive. This is most especially true of the study groups—but find one if you can that functions on its own and is not a franchise of a national organization, as the syllabus provided by such an organization may tend to run along the lines of a Sunday School manual.

Study groups are interesting things. They were started as a means by which homeopaths could find some patients. Since advertising a medical practice was then considered unseemly, the doctors instead would give free lectures in the public library. Or they would sponsor a study group.

To me more to the point, their wives would run the study group, while their husbands—the homeopaths—would sponsor them. Study groups usually met in the homeopath's office, which was usually part of his family home. The homeopath's wife would gather together a group of her husband's patients for a monthly or semi-monthly gathering that was part tea party, part classroom. There they could bring their questions on their own cases, and learn the basics of homeopathic home healthcare, what remedies they should have on hand in their home, how they should store them, how they should use them, and so on.

It was actually a very successful concept. After all, any woman who had lived with a homeopath for a period of years was more than able to instruct on the uses of Arnica, and, if a question was asked that required a more complex answer, well, then the doctor himself could be produced at a moment's notice.

Today, many study groups still are sponsored by individual homeopathic practitioners and still take place in their offices. Many more, however, are run by the laypeople themselves and settle into public places, in libraries, community colleges, churches, and the like, and have evolved into a pure education in homeopathy itself, as they do not have as their purpose either the building of an individual practice or the selling of remedies. With the money motive removed, they are free to get down to the business of education.

In some parts of the country where there are still no practitioners to be found, the study groups can even take the place of the homeopaths. The members of the group can turn to each other for help and advice. Together they can work through a case and solve it.

If you are intent in learning as much about homeopathy as you can, then you are going to have to find yourself a study group. Check community calendars. Call holistic centers. Call doctors' offices. If all else fails, start one yourself. The only important rule of thumb to remember is never to pretend that you know more than you do and never, ever try to work beyond your skill level. If the best you can do is to give information on Arnica and how it helped your five year old when he fell down on the playground, then stick to that. Today, there are so many tapes, books, and other educational materials available on the subject of homeopathy that there is simply no reason that you can't join or form a study group. And as this will be the place in which you will likely receive your best education in homeopathy, it is certainly worth whatever effort it takes to get the studying going.

You may even find that it will be so satisfying and keep you so busy that you glance up from your work one day and find that fifteen years have passed.

After that, like me, you may finally put your feet up and decide that it is someone else's turn.

PART THREE

Healing

"What is impossible for mortals is possible for God."
—THE GOSPEL OF LUKE 18:27

"That which does not kill me only makes me stronger."
—FRIEDRICH NIETZSCHE

CHAPTER NINETEEN

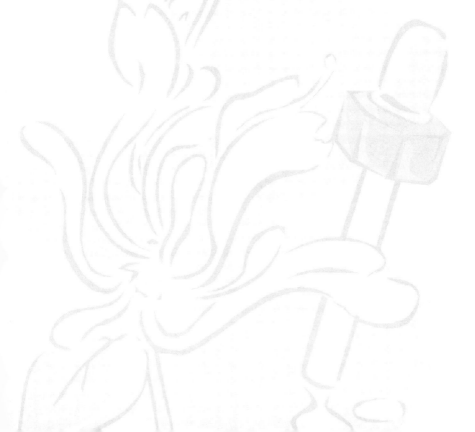

Striking the Match

Because I have never made much money from teaching people about homeo-pathy, I have had to have any number of jobs along the way. And because I loved to teach, it seemed natural at some point that I would work with children within the classroom setting.

So I did.

For a number of years, I worked in the gifted program in the public schools. For those of you who went to school after our government decided that it was no longer cost effective to try to help gifted students to develop their gifts, let me say that, at one point in our history, students who had been identified as being gifted, either through skills testing or general IQ tests, spent part of their school day developing their particular skills. I was assigned to work with those who had been designated as being "high verbal." In other words, potential actors, writers, journalists, and others who were likely to one day make their living through the spoken or written word.

As a product of these programs, I knew just what a waste of time they could be. I had spent countless hours of class time in my own "gifted" program (we called it "high track" in those days) sitting in a room with a few other misfits while a speed-reading machine shot words across the classroom wall. In this way, we speed-read classic nov-els and textbooks and were then tested to see how much information we had absorbed. Those who absorbed the most were considered the most gifted.

Perhaps it was because of this experience that I decided, when it was suddenly my turn to teach, that I wanted to work more directly with the students, from the time of their being identified as "gifted" onward. Therefore, after a few months of just taking the students assigned to me, I decided to take a more active role and I spent a good many hours in the general classroom talking with the students and testing them in their verbal skills instead of relying upon their regular classroom teachers to identify their gifted students themselves.

This made for a profound change in just who filled the seats in the gifted classroom. Where I had before found myself facing a room full of very tidy students, who sat upright and spoke only when spoken to, I now had a group of angry, messy and, often, smelly students who were only grateful to me because, by choosing them, I got them out of their classrooms.

When I tested the students themselves instead of relying upon their test scores, I found that the truly *gifted* (as opposed to the intelligent or motivated) students were often the ones who were getting low grades and dragging the class down. Sometimes this was simply because they were so bored. Most often it was because their actual gifts made it harder for them to fit in with the group of students with whom they found themselves. And very often the most gifted were those who tested worse than any of the others.

So while the teachers were selecting just who they would send to my room, they were picking their best-behaved students, the ones with high grades and quick minds. And thereby using the gifted program as a rewards program for hard work. This was further enforced by the parents of the motivated students, who saw the gifted program as something that looked particularly good on a school resume and pushed hard for their children to be included, gifted or not.

In my testing, I often found that these motivated students would only spit back at me the information that I had programmed in, while the student in the last row, the one who spent most of her time staring out the window, humming to herself, would often be the one who would process the programmed information and use it or bend it in a new way. That, to me, is what gifted is all about.

Now this is a very long way around to make a simple point: healing comes into our lives just as gifts and talents do. It is born into us, whether we ask for it or not. And it often doesn't show up on any tests.

Healing is an animal thing. It is a sloppy thing. It is more often the product of tears and terror than it is of cool, white rooms, and smooth hands brushing their polished nails against fevered brows. Like any other natural process, it is a smelly thing, a pulsing thing. And, like any other natural process, we kid ourselves both as individuals and as a society if we pretend that we can fully understand and tame this process.

The Healing Process

From the moment of birth until the moment of death, healing is always a part of our lives. In that each new moment brings myriad new experiences and catalysts, and in that we do not, with each new stressor, become ill, we can know that healing is an ongoing organic process, always with us, like breathing, like digestion. It is a natural, permanent part of *self*. It is a part of our learning process and of our personal evolution. And it is a fundamental requirement of life.

Throughout that period between birth and death we are always living in some aspect of this process of healing. Sometimes to a greater extent, sometimes to a lesser extent. Sometimes with great success, and sometimes with no apparent success at all.

The problem with our truly understanding the nature of our healing process is the fact that it is invisible and intangible. For scientists, it is as thorny a problem as is the origin of and maintenance of life itself. We know that to sustain our lives, we have to eat, sleep, and breathe. We have to be housed in a manner that protects us and we have to never run with scissors. Our experience of life tells us that we have to also maintain some mechanism within that allows us to interact with our environment, from viruses to grizzly bears, and adapt successfully within it. In other words, we have to attain and maintain an ability to heal.

As I have said before, medicine works with the goal of curing, not healing. This is because as an external and objective process, curing can be measured, and, to some extent, replicated in the lives of any number of patients, all with the same situation requiring cure.

Healing, therefore—irrational, subjective, and internal as it is—takes us outside and beyond the realm of medicine, both homeopathic and allopathic, while it still, at the same time, remains the mechanism that doctors depend upon in order to achieve their cures.

You would think that doctors of all sorts, therefore, would want to know all that they can about the healing process, and would do all that they could to encourage it. But this most certainly is not the case. Most medical professionals of all stripes are trained to seek only the cure, measure only the cure and not to enter into the realm of healing at all, as this is largely seen as the domain of religious and not medical personnel. That's how we end up with cardiologists who don't know enough to ask about a patient's diet, while they are highly skilled in the use of their technological tools. The aspects of life that are rooted to the innate healing process are the aspects that might be considered to be "animal things," those basic parts of life—eating, breathing, sleeping. Because our doctors have removed themselves from the animal, in search of the scientist—who is, in their view, far removed from the animal—they have removed themselves from the aspects of life that are required in order for us to heal. They therefore do not understand the fundamentals of healing and remain puzzled when their cures go awry. And, as doctors seem less and less willing to enter the pit with their patients, the pit of that patient's suffering, as they become less and less willing to cry with their patients as their patients wrestle with their disease, the same doctors become less and less able to help their patients stir up their healing process and use it to help them to evolve past their disease.

As the medical process becomes ever more one of diagnosis and treatment, followed by failure or success, and then followed by an endless repetition of the same, the patient—as a sweaty animal being—is lost, the doctor as another animal, one called along side to help and protect, is lost, and, in the mix, the patient's healing potential is also lost. Thrown out the window for the sake of the pretense that we have evolved beyond the very thing we need to be in order to heal. As the practice of medicine becomes as sterile as its workrooms, this factory-timed process of diagnosis/treatment, diagnosis/treatment, diagnosis/treatment can only result in more and more failure than success.

And when the best that you can say about a treatment is that the patient managed to withstand it and get well in spite of it, then we are indeed approaching the point at which all hope is lost.

The healing process is an animal process. Machines do not and cannot heal. To take the human hand out of the healing interplay between doctor and patient and to replace it with the touch of metal is to drain the possibility of healing out of the encounter. In the same way, to take away a natural healing substance and to replace it with a chemical substitute in the name of "safety" and "control" (terms that are used in place of the actual reason, which is a matter of branding and owning that which belongs to all), is to take something that speaks to us and to our potential for healing within the same framework within which we live and thrive and to replace it with something artificial, something that can only attempt to replicate the power of the original.

If our medical science is going to abandon this issue of healing, then it is incumbent upon us to understand healing in our own lives and in the lives of those we love. We have to become as skilled as we can in methods that can encourage our process of healing in every moment of our lives, most especially in the times of a health crisis. We have to, in a very real way, become physicians for ourselves and for those in our lives.

Poison Ivy

Young or old, rich or poor, male or female, we each of us have within us an amazing ability to heal.

Take me for example. If I have any expertise when it comes to health and healing it comes hard earned. As I look back over my fifty years of life, I can see, fading off into the distance, an almost endless number of illnesses. Some I would say I dealt with very successfully, others, less so. And yet, in spite of them all, I am still here. I have managed to maintain my life and health, and, with work and struggle, to improve them, often against all medical belief and hope.

The list of my ailments is long—colitis, migraine, allergies of all sorts, chronic fatigue, hypertension, hemorrhages, and endless numbers of respiratory infections, to name a few.

If we can equate a large number of illnesses over a long period of time with a weakness in terms of healing, and if we can equate illness with vulnerability on a fundamental level, then I am a very vulnerable being. And in that I have been beset with allergies, which are nothing more than a healing system gone paranoid, in that it reacts, or overreacts, to benign aspects of the environment, then my healing process is overactive. And in that I have a history of many, many upper respiratory infections, infections that would most often last much longer in my body than in the bodies of everyone else around me, it has to also be concluded that I have an underactive healing mechanism. All in all, not a very good success story.

But, over the years, as I succumbed to illness after illness, there has always been poison ivy, and, sometimes, poison ivy has been all that has gotten me through.

You see, I am not allergic to poison ivy at all. You can roll me in it, feed it to me, and I won't get it. I never have, not once in fifty years. I have a sister who is terribly allergic to it, and gets it every year, from the top of her head to the bottom of her feet. She has had it inside her body as well as out. To see her suffer from poison ivy is a terrible thing.

But here we are with the same parents, from the same gene pool, and she's vulnerable and I'm immune.

Now, is the ivy less poison when it comes around me? Is the corrosive liquid that the plant produces less corrosive when I touch it than when my sister does? Of course not. But it is less corrosive where I am concerned. The catalyst of the plant elicits no response from me.

And, in the same way, we have found patients who should have AIDS, but do not, although they have the HIV virus present in their body. And it is the same with every other disease. For every deadly condition there is someone who just does not feel the effects of this condition as he should.

> . . . our inborn ability to heal is far more powerful, and far more dependable, than any form of medicine ever could hope to be.

To me this is a profound thing. I can't get past the thought that, if it is within the realm of human possibility for any given disease to be resisted or healed, then it is within the realm of possibility for *me* to be resistant to it or healed from it. In the same way, while each of us is vulnerable to some things, there are other conditions—sometimes those that are quite deadly to almost everyone else—to which we are quite invulnerable, like Superman with bullets bouncing off. Whether we look at the healing process on an individual level or as an innate power of the species, the power to heal is an awesome thing.

Given that while a disease may kill some of the people all of the time, and all of the people some of the time, but no disease can kill all of the people all of the time, our inborn ability to heal is far more powerful, and far more dependable, than any form of medicine ever could hope to be.

The Power of Possibility

By this, I do not mean to imply that medicine—especially homeopathic medicine—used appropriately cannot be a true healing tool. I know that in my own life, I have become much stronger, much less prone to illness and much quicker to heal, through the use of homeopathic medicine.

But I also know that there are other tools, some just as vital as the remedies, which can be used to produce a healing result.

The mind, for example, is a potent tool for healing. And a way in which the mind can be harnessed to work toward healing is by presenting the mind with the *possibility* of healing.

Try this technique. It can be a great help to anyone who is suffering from any form of illness, acute or chronic, although I have seen it work most powerfully with those who have been worn down by long-term illnesses. It is especially helpful to those with pain.

Ask the patient, or ask yourself if you are the one in pain, "Do you believe that it is possible for you to not have this pain?" By this, you are asking if it exists at all within the realm of possibility. If there is one chance in a million that they could be free of the pain. And by free of the pain, I mean free of that pain for only a brief time. Perhaps only for a second.

What you are trying to do is open the door to the possibility that they could be free of the pain, or of any other symptom or symptoms. That they could be whole again, if only for a second.

If the patient feels that there is no possibility of their being pain free, even only for a moment, then reduce the challenge again and ask if in their wildest imagination such a thing could occur. If they cannot picture it in reality, then let them picture it on Mars or in any other place that can occur to them. But find the place, the time, and the circumstance in which the possibility of healing can occur.

When you finally move from a "no" to a "yes" then you can move forward with the technique in the same way that you would if the patient had agreed to the possibility of being pain free when first asked. Help them create that circumstance in their mind.

Ask again, "Is it possible for you to be pain free?" When they say yes, ask, "Could you let go of your pain right now, for just one moment?"

Again, you are seeking a positive response. The next step is to ask, "Would you let go of your pain right now, for just one second?"

When they feel that they not only can be free of pain but that they are also willing to be free of the pain, then you have only to say, "Let it go."

Look at what happens next.

Watch the patient's face. Some will yawn, others will sigh, and still others will laugh. All of these things are signs of release.

If there is no release, you may have to try again. You may have to try again and again. In some cases, patients will feel a marked improvement from simply letting go of the pain, a moment at a time. In other cases, the patient may have greater difficulty releasing their pain.

Either way, the technique is a process. It is not a pill. But it allows the patient's mind to begin to wrestle with the possibility that they can indeed be healed, that they can release their pain and be free of their disease.

A great deal has been written about creative imagery. About helping the patient to take himself from his bed within his mind's eye and to place himself in the green pastures promised in the twenty-third Psalm. Some imagine a white light flooding the diseased part of their body. Others imagine their immune system rising up as a literal army and striking down all the diseased cells in their path. All of these visualizations can be powerful healing tools, because they all allow for the possibility of healing.

In the name of informed consent, so many medical practitioners inflict so much harm on their patients. Patients have to hear terrible news of upcoming pain and, possibly, death from the lips of a person who has been culturally established as being one in almost ultimate authority. The obvious danger in this is one of self-fulfilling prophecy. The patient who leaves their doctor's office in a state of confusion and fear has left that office weaker and more likely to lose their battle with their disease than they were before they walked in. And, sadly, so often the information that is presented as if it were scientific fact and totally incontrovertible is, in all reality only one practitioner's opinion. At best, it is the product of a mortal mind that, for all its attempts at understanding the nature of health and disease, really hasn't much more than a series of hunches and observations to go on. At worst, the dreaded diagnosis may just be the babbling of a fool in a white lab coat.

Any doctor who removes the possibility of healing from his patients' minds is, in my opinion, not involved with the practice of medicine, but with its malpractice.

Medical professionals of all sorts and stripes need to constantly remind themselves that in every moment they must do all that they can to elevate the mind of their patient. And to increase in their thoughts the possibility they might be healed.

Use the technique. Try it on yourself next time you are ill. Create the possibility for healing. Allow for the fact that you can just let the pain go. Only for a second at first. Then perhaps for a longer period of time.

In the same way, perhaps healing will only be a remote possibility at first. But with time and with repeated attempts at releasing the pain that possibility can become a probability. So that you can at last ask, "Do you think that it is probable that you will be healed?" And that the response is a direct "yes." Then you can be sure that the healing process has begun.

With this simple technique, and others like it, you can enlist the power of the human mind as a tool for healing. But there is a tool for healing that I believe is ever more powerful—the human spirit.

The Power of Assertion

Along this line of thinking, I remember that many years ago, I was once reading a book on homeopathy while I was a passenger in a car that was traveling from Connecticut up to Martha's Vineyard in Massachusetts.

Now, in those years, I was always reading books on homeopathy. Often I would want to read aloud from them to everyone else in the car. But in that they had all had experience with me reading about blood, pus, and stool quality, my friends had long since insisted that I not read aloud under any circumstances.

That day, the book I was reading was *The Science of Homeopathy* by George Vithoulkas. Now without any doubt, Vithoulkas is one of the modern masters of the art of practicing homeopathy. And this book is one of the greatest works of homeopathic literature. But, oh, that word "science"—right there in the title. That word for me is such a bitter pill to swallow. But I was determined, after having read another of Vithoulkas's books, that I would get through this one.

To say that this book was not an easy read for me is putting in mildly. Tolstoy, in comparison, was an easy, fun read. I had already in my young life made it through the *Lord of the Rings* twice, with its endless descriptions of what the hobbits were having for dinner, but this book was making my head hurt and the motion of the moving car wasn't making things any easier.

Then I read a short passage that has stayed with me ever since. That passage, on page 90 of the book, read: "The 'laying on of hands' by a highly evolved spiritual individual is another therapy which can directly affect the plane of the electromagnetic field.... 'Laying on of hands' by a spiritually evolved person who is in fact a channel for universal energies can directly strengthen the defense mechanism and thereby bring about a lasting cure. The drawback to this is that there will always be too few people of such spiritual evolution to effectively deal with the health problems of our age."

This from the man who fills his pages with Venn diagrams and flow charts? This from the man who writes sentences so dense, so convoluted as to make Henry James blush? All of a sudden there was talk of faith healing and "universal energies"?

It simply amazes me that, in this text on science and homeopathic healing—a book whose sole goal is trying to convince me that homeopathy actually *is* scientific—that there is this expressed belief that something as irrational and nonscientific as laying on of hands can result in healing. Or in what the author calls "a lasting cure."

With this brief passage, one in which the author concludes on page 98 that "three modes of therapy are capable of acting directly on the dynamic plane: acupuncture, 'laying on of hands' by a spiritually evolved individual, and homeopathy," Vithoulkas opens the door wide to a consideration of the power of assertion, which is to say, the power of prayer.

After all, that actual physical touch—the laying on of the hands in "laying on of hands"—is merely a point of contact between the object of prayer and the person—that "spiritually evolved individual"—asserting the truth. That healing is not only possible, but also the correct functioning of the universe. That what we call miraculous is, in reality, the normal flow of events.

For me, prayer is all about assertion, and assertion, if harnessed correctly, is all about prayer.

Prayer is also about belief, of course. Belief in God is the wellspring of prayer. And there will be more about the power of belief in a moment, belief on the part of the patient and of the healer as well. But for the moment, let's consider assertion.

I come from the Christian tradition, and so can only have an understanding of healing in that tradition. But each religious philosophy contains both the concept of faith healing and the procedure to be followed in times of need. In the New Testament, we are told that, when we are ill, we are to summon the elders of the church for laying on of hands.

To read these Scriptures is to understand that, for those who lived in times in which they were written, the procedure of praying for the sick was far more than a second thought, more than something that the family could do while they were barred from the patient's hospital room. No, to these people prayer was medicine and this was the acceptable procedure for dealing with those in a health crisis. What we would today think of as medicine—a specific herbal remedy, a poultice, tincture, or rub—would have been the second thought in terms of treatment, if it had been used at all.

In the two thousand years of modern human history, we have seen a slow march away from spirituality in medicine and toward a scientific approach. And, somehow, the term "scientific" has taken on the connotation of being superior as a methodology to all others, including the spiritual. Instead of realizing that there are many methods of thinking, many approaches to life in general and to health and healing specifically, the scientific mind can recognize only one—its own.

The problem with this, with putting all our eggs in the one cart of scientific methodology—which is to say, trial and error—is that the scientific method of discovery yields conclusions that are ever-changing. That which was healthful for us yesterday is today found to be harmful. Healing drugs are discovered to be killer drugs, or vice versa, with each new study. And to understand the truth and ramifications of each study, we have to explore not only its mode of information gathering, but also the source of its funding and their particular interest in the given study's outcome.

If we lived in a world in which pure science was allowed to exist and scientists were encouraged (or even allowed) to seek the truth no matter what that truth may do to an individual corporate interest, then perhaps we could have a means of developing a system of technological medicine that was itself hale and hearty. But we live in a world in which business interests and government funding to a large part determine not only exactly what is studied, but, to some lesser or greater extent, the outcome of the studies themselves. That can only lead us to question just how healthy our medical system itself can be if it is based on information that just can't be fully trusted.

Prayer, on the other hand, supersedes the functioning of modern medicine. Prayer allows us to express our assurance that there is more to us than meat and bones. And that our invisible nature, whatever you want to call it, is the more important part of our being. The part that is eternal in nature. Further, prayer allows us to communicate with an intelligence far greater than that of any individual human, even one who graduated from the Yale School of Medicine.

I do believe that we live in a universe that is most eager to please. I believe that the reality that we physically experience is to some extent determined by our expectations of it. In this setting, I believe that prayer can help determine reality. There is power in assertion, power in prayer.

Perhaps we have made a mistake in removing prayer from our standard of what is considered traditional and acceptable in medical care. Perhaps we need to develop a new model that speaks to our invisible as well as our visible nature.

Given all that I have already written, I guess that it would be foolish of me to note that scientific studies have indeed concluded the efficacy of prayer in healing the sick. But unless these studies were paid for by Catholic charities, perhaps they can be trusted.

The Power of Belief

I may be splitting hairs to separate prayer and belief. As I have already said, the very foundation of prayer *is* belief, but that belief is specific to the existence of a deity of some sort, whether that being be perceived as a benevolent father or, more vaguely, as some sore of "universal intelligence." Wrestling with that belief, or lack thereof, is part of the riddle of prayer. Can we pray with our whole hearts if we just plain don't believe that anyone is listening? That is for each individual to decide. And, in making that decision, it is for each person to decide whether or not the act of prayer is appropriate.

But here I am talking about a different sort of belief, one that may or may not connect to a personal religious commitment.

This is a simple belief—one that connects back to that idea of the power of possibility.

Time and again I have seen that, in order for the sick to be made well, someone has to believe that it is possible for them to be made well. If all agree—doctor, nurses, loved ones, and patient—that the case is hopeless, then the patient will die. In all cases of illnesses, and most especially in cases of chronic or life-threatening illness, it is vitally important that

> In all cases of illnesses, and most especially in cases of chronic or life-threatening illness, it is vitally important that the belief of healing be encouraged, be allowed to spark and ignite.

the belief of healing be encouraged, be allowed to spark and ignite.

Now this does not mean that the patient himself has to believe that he can be healed. I have seen many patients who have given up on themselves, only to have a loved one, a wife, or parent or friend, anchor them back in the world with the power of belief. And sometimes when all the world has given up on the patient, he himself from his hospital bed will simply refuse to give up on this belief and will turn a bad situation around. I have also seen many caregivers sit by their patient's bed, knowing against all scientific evidence, that that patient can get well.

Someone somewhere in that chain of care and support has got to keep the belief of healing alive. There is tremendous power in this belief, and tremendous harm is done to patients who are given scientific fact in the guise of universal truth. Like insurance agents deciding who to insure and not insure, too many of our doctors have become skilled at playing the odds and have forgotten that each patient is a whole and unique being. In looking at each new patient, that doctor is, in all reality not just looking at the next case of the same old clump of symptoms, but is, instead, looking at something that he has never seen before—something completely new who will react to illness and healing and treatment in a manner that is completely different from anyone else he has ever seen or treated.

Each of us deserves the right to be treated as a whole and unique being. And each of us needs to have someone who believes that healing is possible if healing is to take place.

The Power of Desire

This last part's the hardest to discuss, and, often, the hardest to overcome. But sometimes you just want to look into the eyes of a patient, especially one who is seriously ill, or who has been ill for a long, long time and ask, "Do you want to be well?"

Now everyone will insist that they want nothing more than to be totally well. But, often this is just not the truth. We live in a society that, in my opinion, actually encourages us to get sick and rewards us for staying sick.

For many of us, the only time we really get attention is when we are ill. Little children learn early on that, when they are sick, they get to stay in bed and their mother will fuss over them and make them soup. In the same way, many millions of senior citizens find themselves invisible in society and find that they are literally untouched, unhugged, and unwanted until they make an appointment at a doctor's office. These same seniors will often speak of their doctor as if he were their best friend. And why not, here is someone who pays attention to them, asks them questions and listens to their answers, looks at them, touches them and seems genuinely concerned about whether or not they live or die. Further, the doctor offers them an office in which they are greeted by the receptionist, the nurses, and the office staff, which is far more than they get at the grocery store or at Wal-Mart. We have allowed our doctors' offices, at least for this growing segment of our society, to become a hub of social activity.

So, from childhood to old age, and in all the years in between, we have been conditioned to believe that illness brings us a certain set of entitlements, special attention, special foods, all geared to making our suffering a little less and our lives a little happier. But the conditioning doesn't stop there.

We also have our television sets and those damned commercials for pharmaceuticals again. On these ads, the people who take their purple pills get to go on picnics and swing on swings. Their lives are full and happy, and the implication here is that this is not just due to the fact that, with the purple pill, they are pain free, but that the very taking of that pill will make them better to be around.

Worse still is an advertisement that I've recently noticed for selling prescription drugs with the notion that, by having a chronic disease, you have somehow joined a club or an organization. In these ads, illnesses are not called by names, but by friendlier abbreviations. Thus, rheumatoid arthritis, a very painful condition, is called "RA" And all the folks with RA get to hang around together and take their medication and suppress their pain and go on a picnic together.

I mean, come on, does it take a genius to realize that it is completely counterproductive to healing, to actually getting over rheumatoid arthritis, to give the disease a happy name and form a club around living with it? Does it take a genius to realize that this might have more to do with the fact that if drug companies can produce medications that control symptoms they can make a good deal more money than they would if they produced medications that actually cured those symptoms?

There's this great old movie called "The Man in the White Suit" starring Alec Guinness. It's a great old British comedy. In the movie, Alec Guinness invents a pure white suit that is made of an indestructible material. It cannot be stained or ruined. When word gets out of this discovery, there are business interests that will stop at nothing to make sure that this suit disappears and that no other suits are ever made.

Arguments are made that the economy would be ruined if a perfect suit were ever made. In the same way, the drug companies must truly fear the idea of medicine that actually works, because that would result in their selling a lot less medicine.

Fact is, we are living in a world in which we are more valuable as consumers than we are as human beings.

And let's also face the fact that we are quite simply fools if we allow ourselves to be convinced that we should take our consumer medical advice from television commercials. They exist only to sell a product and in no way are concerned with our health as individual beings, or, for that matter, the safety and efficacy of the product sold. Taking medical advice from commercial television makes about as much sense as going into marital counseling with Lucille Ball and Desi Arnaz.

The point is that we have created a culture that so strongly encourages us to live our lives with a series of "controllable" illnesses—ailments that will to some extent limit our lives for the rest of our lives, and will require us to buy multiple prescription drugs each month for the rest of our lives, but never quite kill us, or at least not kill us for a few years—that it can take a great deal of effort to even begin to turn that process around.

If you have already used homeopathic medicines in your own life to treat something more serious than a cold or flu, think about how hard it was to make that decision. Especially if you made that decision for an underage child or a beloved pet, for someone or something that you love with all your heart and whose fate was in your hands. Think of all the people that, had they known what you were considering doing, would have at the very least advised you as to how foolish you were being.

And this was just a decision to try another form of medicine, one that grew from the same medical traditions and philosophies as modern allopathy did.

What if you decided not to treat medically at all? What if you decided that prayer constituted medical treatment in and of itself?

Anyone who has ever stepped outside the realm of what is considered culturally to be appropriate and safe medical treatment learns very quickly their reputation changes from upright to intellectually inferior or morally corrupt.

In a medical emergency, when you may not get a second chance at selecting a mode of treatment, it can take all the courage you can muster to decide against the antibiotics or the steroids, or the cold, confusion, noise, and glare of the emergency room. Even in the moments when the danger is not so great, it can be a very difficult thing to move homeopathic philosophy from the written page and enact it in flesh.

All of which takes us back to that original, essential question: "Do you want to be well?"

This question demands of the patient a far deeper and more far-reaching conclusion than the question of homeopathy versus allopathy ever will. It is just as possible to become a homeopathic junkie as it is an allopathic junkie. And entirely too many of today's homeopathic practitioners are just as happy to have you come to their office again and again, pay them again and again for their time and attention and "expertise."

No, there has to be a deeper decision made. One that supersedes the desire to make a doctor's appointment just to be seen, to be recognized as a human being who is *worth* treating.

I have seen it time and again. When the patient decides that he wants to be well, fundamentally wants to be able to live his life, however long that might be, with a sense of freedom of action and creative involvement, then that patient begins instinctively to do the things that will make them well.

Until that decision gets made, the fat patient won't diet, the sad patient will sit alone in his room with his own nagging thoughts, and the weak patient still will eat only tea and toast.

Someone must look into each patient's eyes and ask, "Do you want to be well?" And that person must care about the answer, because, on the level of healing (as opposed to curing) the answer to that question determines most of what is to follow.

The Movement toward Healing

Declaring that the bond between the patient and his illness is cultural—the product of television advertising and mother love—is just too easy, I know. It in no way describes the intricacy of that bond, the many ways in which the patient can have his life defined for him by his illness. The ways in which illness can set the standard of life and the rules by which it will be lived. And, on the deepest level, what intimate things that our illnesses can whisper to us about ourselves. Symptoms—especially the symptoms of chronic debilitating conditions—can be Loreleis, luring us all to steer our ships to the reef. Or illness can be like joining the army—a system that will tell you when to get up, when to go to bed, and what to do with the time between. It can make for a life simplified—a life in which your purpose and goal can become a very simple thing indeed—just coping with your disease.

It can be a very difficult thing indeed to decide that you want to become well if your illness is what is getting you up in the morning, what is forcing you to eat if you do not want to eat, if only so that you can take your pills. The reality is, for millions of us, we just would not know what we would do *without* our illnesses, what our lives might be. It is one thing to consider the young person who suddenly becomes ill. If they are made well, if they can just experience the absence of that illness, then their lives are long and their bodies are strong. But, for the middle-aged person with hypertension and diabetes, or the elderly person with a plethora of ills, what can they suspect their lives would be without their illness? Millions of us, I believe, have become so used to our illnesses that they have become like mates that we no longer love, certainly don't hate, and keep us from facing life alone. The hollow existence that enters into so many of our relationships also enters our own bodies in the form of our health. I believe that on a fundamental, unknowable level, we have accepted the health system we have—one that offers maintenance of poor health instead of healing—because we don't really want to be completely well. The person in a complete state of health is, after all, in a complete state of freedom of movement and creativity. In other words, all excuses are gone. This means, on the surface level, that "I can't exercise because of my back" simply has got to go. And on a deeper level it means that, as we are told in the Scriptures, to whom much is given, much is required.

In truth, health—a great gift—brings with it a great responsibility. And we are therefore quite lucky that we have such cooperative bodies that will break down for us just when we want an excuse to stay in bed.

The decision to become healthy is, therefore, not nearly as simple a thing as it seems. It means that we are going to have to go through a divorce of sorts. We are going to have to divorce our old ways, our old habits, and, hardest of all, our old thoughts. If we want to be well then we have to first accept the fact that our innate power to heal ourselves is far more powerful than we might want it to be. We have to accept the fact that our illnesses are something more than the luck of the genetic draw.

Homeopathy offers a healing tool, as does acupuncture and as does the laying on of hands. Perhaps there are other pure tools for healing as well. The point here is not to list them, but to remind us that they are merely tools. That nothing, no medicine or tool, will be able to create a process of healing if our system will not itself enter into a state of healing. Medicine can, I believe, offer cures that require no permission, no agreement on the part of the patient, which can leave the patient, after an operation or some other potent means of forcing a cure, in the rather ironic state of being cured but not healed, not whole.

I spent the majority of this book first talking about medicine and then about homeopathic medicine specifically, trying to compare and contrast the two, one the subset of the other, as they attempt to bring about a cure.

In these last few pages, I write not about curing anything, not about what remedy to give when the patient has a specific set of symptoms, but about something more difficult still. Something that is taking place along side of this struggle to cure. Something that may happen in spite of a failure to cure. And, finally, something that is much more important to the life and possible death of a patient than whether or not they are ultimately cured. And that, of course, is healing.

In all the various flavors of medicine, we can happily limit the need for a cure to something that only sick people need. And we never quite get around to dealing with just where the line is between sickness and health—what it is that makes a con-dition bearable for one person, but sends another person for help. Our doctors of all kinds tend to just sort of wait passively for the patients to self-identify their need. If they show up with money or an insurance card, then they are given treatment, which is to say, medicine.

This is the system that we have in place. It is one that does not address in any way the need for healing.

So, then, with a limited health system, a cultural bond with managed chronic ill-nesses of all sorts and our own quiet complicity with disease, how do we begin the movement toward healing in our own life and in the lives of those we love?

First by acknowledging that we can do it. We are capable of healing more power-fully and more completely than we ever seem to allow.

That means that we do, on some level, have to make a decision to be well. We do have to decide to take charge, to no longer let the disease dictate the situation. And, ironically, it means that in the moment in which we are weakest—when we are in pain, in fear, or in danger of our lives—we are going to have to be our strongest as well.

That suggests the second stage, which is the decision to risk it. In the movie "Out of Africa," there is a wonderful line that says that the world is round so that we cannot "see too far down the road." The decision to work toward healing is one that must be made in spite of what one might find down the road. Further, it is a decision that must be made today and again tomorrow and the day after and the day after that. As a process, it must not only be committed to, but also committed to again and again, most especially as the hard times come and as the battles appear to be lost.

The third part of this process involves then doing something about it. That may mean going to a homeopath and working with him as he attempts to bring about a homeopathic cure. That may also mean that you will have to change your diet, your lifestyle, and your thought process. There is no one map to success. After all, if you can accept that in illness you are a unique being who experiences illness in a unique manner, then, in healing, you must surely be willing to accept that your path to heal-ing will be yours and yours alone.

The important thing is, that as you work to become both well and whole, you do it every day. Do something every day that will move you to health and freedom. If you can't move your leg, then try to move your toe. Every day. There are no days of rest here in the healing process. I state the obvious, but, just as I have written above that the mind and the spirit must be used as tools for healing, I now point out that the body must be used in this way as well. So many people who are sick just ignore the things that we all know we need to do in order to be well—breathing correctly, sleeping deeply, drinking enough water, eating the right foods, and so forth.

The point is simply this: if there are three levels of being—body, mind, and spirit—then when healing is required it is required by all three and will in turn require all three levels to work together in the healing process. Nothing else is going to work. To pretend that you, as a whole being, can just cure your body and your mind and spirit will putter along as they have before is to return to the allopathic simplistic hope that a disease can be separated from the patient with the disease, almost without them noticing. As if a cure can be imposed with no ramifications.

Keep in mind that there is a distinction between healing and curing. Never confuse the two. Never sell yourself or those you love short by accepting a cure when a healing is in order.

Remember, we can cure without healing or heal without curing. Sadly, we can fail at both as well. But, in the best result, we can both be cured and healed. We can not only let go of the physical, mental, and emotional ravages of disease, but we can also be made whole, be made free, and made powerful.

> Remember, we can cure without healing or heal without curing. . . . But, in the best result, we can both be cured and healed.

Medicine in all its forms will always and only be capable of attempts at curing. That is all it can and will ever do. But we ourselves, in our hearts and minds and spirits, are capable of true healing. We can completely change the rules that have ordered our lives and the lives of those around us. We can set ourselves free, and, in doing so, free all those around us who have had to live with the burden and the restrictions of our illness.

Think for a moment of a time in which you have been ill—acutely or chronically—and what that meant in the lives of those around you. The stresses in their lives that your illness created. The modifications your illness required in their lifestyles, in their creative enjoyment of life. It is very difficult to accomplish much in your own life if you are having to pour your life energy into the needs of the person you love. This is the whirlpool effect of illness. Even in the case of one person and one ailment, it touches and distorts so many lives.

The Ripple Effect

Healing, on the other hand, has a ripple effect all its own. It touches so many people and leaves them better for having been touched.

The transformation, in moving from illness to health, is from Consumer to Creator.

Our celebrities tell us, as they cut the ribbon on a new hospital wing, that they are just "giving back" to their community. This, of course, implies some sort of success on their part that allows them to give. They give because they have surplus.

The sick, especially the dangerously sick or the chronically sick, have no surpluses. They consume the stockpiles they have set aside or from the stockpiles of others.

In a successful move from sickness to health, the patient finds himself once more able to create surplus, in energy, in thought, in possessions. And this surplus once more allows him to give of himself and his bounty. This is the ripple effect. The one who so needed embracing for so long can now once more return the embrace. This is the natural outcome of the healing process.

Remember, to whom much has been given, much is required.

And that is just as it should be.

CHAPTER TWENTY

Lighting the Fire

J ust one thing more, and then we're done.

It is important if you are going to be of any help to anyone in a health crisis that you first place yourself in a position to be capable of offering real help. This may mean that before you can reach out and help others you must first heal yourself.

Now I know that in a crisis, especially a crisis that involves a loved one being in danger or in pain, your first instinct may be to try and take a heroic action that will put things right. But until you yourself are centered and ready to take that action, you will not only not be of any use, you may actually do a great deal of harm. If you are too emotionally involved in the situation and find that you cannot get to the place within yourself that you can think clearly and act appropriately, then you must move aside and let others take action in your place. If the situation at hand is one beyond your ability to treat appropriately—if you know nothing more about home-opathy than the use of a handful of "household" remedies, and your husband is hav-ing a heart attack—then you must summon appropriate help. Indeed, in all cases of life-threatening health crises, the appropriate first step is to call for emergency med-ical assistance. If, while waiting for help to arrive, you have the skill to palliate symp-toms or to actually turn the crises around with an appropriate remedy, then so much the better. But there is, in my opinion, nothing quite so dangerous as an unskilled student of homeopathy working beyond their depth in an emotionally charged and physically dangerous situation.

Luckily, it is much more common that the health crisis at hand will be far less threatening—for example an acute ailment like cold or flu or a simple mechanical injury. These things are far easier to treat, both in terms of the actual threat to the overall health of the patient and to the emotional health of the person who is, by the circumstances, required to take on the physician's role.

And in taking on that role, always remember the roles required in the formation of any healing team. In order to take on the physician's role, you must be able to get to the place of being compassionately objective. One whose job it is to both gather needed information and to act with the intent of bringing about a true cure. To get the job done and the case cured, you need to have that functioning healing team in place. The keyword there is "functioning."

And here's how to make sure that it is functioning as it should.

Before making use of your homeopathic kit, you may need to take a remedy yourself. You may need Arnica for trauma or Aconite for shock, depending upon the circumstances of the crisis at hand. Or you may need the support of a Bach flower remedy like Rescue Remedy or Star of Bethlehem before you can function with a clear mind. Or you may just need to take ten seconds for yourself and remind yourself of what your function is here. But before you do anything for the patient, make sure that you do take those few seconds first to be sure that you are capable of enacting the role of the physician and all that that implies.

Functioning in a Crisis

Above all else, your primary function is to do nothing that will inhibit the patient's own ability to heal. This is true on all levels. The patient should no more receive a psychic trauma from you in the form of fear or despair than he should receive a poison from you in the place of a medicine. Remember that this single goal, this "first do no harm" has two parts when put into action. While you are seeking to bring about a cure with the wise and appropriate use of homeopathic remedies, you are, at the same time, also trying to create circumstances in which the patient's own healing mechanism will work to its best ability. Remember that you are treating a whole being here; you are never treating a list of symptoms.

Your second function is to gather the information you need in order to select an appropriate remedy.

This means that you must begin to assess the situation just as soon as you are ready to do so. Don't just start firing questions at the patient. Instead, witness who they are and how they are acting. Take in all that is happening with all your senses.

No matter the circumstances, it has been my experience that in a crisis situation, you will do better if you can ask as few questions of the patient as possible—indeed, in many circumstances they may not be able to answer your questions—and instead base your drug diagnosis upon the witness of your own senses. If others are present who witnessed the crisis, seek what information you can from them. Then, finally, ask the patient for the information you need in simple, direct questions. But never take your eyes off him. Listen to what he says and watch how he says it. If you have studied well and know your Materia Medica, the patient will communicate with you all that you need to know by their body position, by the strength of their response to stimuli, by their mood, their desires, their fears, and by myriad other ways that they inhabit their situation.

Your second function in terms of information in case taking means that you are going to have to know what to do with that information once you have gathered it. That you are going to have to make the correct drug diagnosis. Given the situation, this may be a very simple thing, such as in the case of a simple mechanical injury in which only a handful of remedies will come to mind as being useful to the patient. Indeed, even some of life's greatest health crises suggest only two or three remedies to differentiate among.

But once you have gathered the needed information on the remedies, you may now face a greater challenge than you have ever faced before. You may have a need of knowledge of the Materia Medica and Repertory that you have never needed before. If your knowledge of Materia Medica is great enough, you may simply know the remedy needed when you see it. If this is not the case, you can still uncover the truth if you know how to take the case apart and repertorize it quickly and effectively. Either way, at this moment your case-taking skills will be your most important tools.

You see, whatever the circumstance, your role remains the same. Always the same. You must objectively decide what changes have taken place through the circumstances of the crisis at hand and then figure out what remedy would create those same symptoms in a well person. This is why I so often say that if you wait until an emergency has already happened, then it is just too late to start studying homeopathy now. All your study of the philosophy of homeopathy, of the Materia Medica, or the Repertory, all of it is geared to this moment. This crisis.

If you have studied well, then in the crisis, you will only have to first center yourself and bring yourself to a mindset in which you can manage to be objective enough to think clearly. Then you will only have to remember two other things. First you will have to remember that this crisis is no different from any other. That the principles by which healing happens are still the same. That the principles by which homeopathic cure happens are still the same. That you need only work through this case like any other and cure will result. And, second, you have to remember to breathe.

Once you have selected the remedy that best speaks to the case, your third function is to manage that case correctly. To not overmedicate the patient, but to stay with them, follow their symptoms as they shift and stay on top of the healing process. Again, don't let your own fear of failure or sense of upset over seeing a loved one in pain tempt you to do things that you should not. Don't let it tempt you to switch from remedy to remedy too often as you thrash about trying to create an improvement. Don't let it tempt you to give a remedy too often or in too high an initial potency in the vain hope that more is indeed better. And don't let it tempt you to mix and match medicines, giving homeopathic, allopathic, and herbal all at once in the hopes that, liked cooked spaghetti, something will stick.

In the moment of crisis, stay the course and know what you know. If you know that homeopathic medicine truly works, then you also know that it works as well in a true crisis as it does when it is being used to combat a toothache or a sty. If you don't know already that homeopathy works, if up until now you have trusted allopathic medicine, then this is not the moment in which you should give something new a try.

And if, in a moment of crisis, in which your own child has a high fever and you feel that you are just too afraid to risk using a remedy instead of getting him the antibiotics that you have seen work in the past, then if you decide in that crisis to give him the antibiotics once more to get him through, then fine, you have made a coherent decision. Once the crisis has passed, once your child is well again and you can think more clearly, then you can work in a new way, learn new skills, and be better prepared to work with a fever in a new way next time, or better still, to strengthen your child's total health so that that next fever is prevented.

The Checklist

So here's a little list. Just some things to consider before you ever treat anyone, before you ever dole out the medicine. I find these questions to be valuable. If I think these through before taking a case, I usually do pretty well. It is the times in which I don't answer these questions honestly, or, worse, the times in which I don't bother to think of these questions at all that I usually get into trouble.

So you might want to think these things through before you take on what is really an awesome responsibility of giving another being any form of medication, any catalyst that might change their life for better or worse for a long time to come. Remember, honesty is a vital component of healing. Just as you need to be able to trust the information given you by your patient and by other witnesses, you have to be able to trust yourself as you enact the role of the physician.

> Remember, honesty is a vital component of healing. Just as you need to be able to trust the information given you by your patient and by other witnesses, you have to be able to trust yourself as you enact the role of the physician.

Before taking a case or treating a patient, ask yourself:

1. If I take this case, am I ready to follow through with it, to stay the course from the beginning until the end?

2. In taking this case, am I willing to work only in the best interest of the patient, and not my own or anyone else's?

3. Am I capable of working with this case successfully? Am I skilled enough to know that I can be of help to the patient?

4. Am I centered in my thinking, calm enough, and thinking clearly enough to be capable of doing good work? Do I need healing myself before proceeding?

5. Am I entering into case taking in an unbiased manner? Am I willing to gather information and use that information appropriately, or have I already formed an opinion about the patient, the case, or the needed remedy?

With these things in mind, do what you now know to do in the manner in which you know to do it. Use whatever doubt or fear or shock you yourself feel to focus your mind and to propel you through the experience. Just don't let that doubt or fear stop you, or persuade you to do something that you know you should not do. Just look for the similarity, find the remedy, decide the potency and dosage, and then wait and look for the change. Work in the moment and keep yourself centered and strong.

You can always fall apart later.

Resources

Following is a listing of books, Internet sites, organizations, pharmacies, and pharmaceutical firms that I can recommend to you as you continue your education in homeopathy. These lists are biased, I admit. Each listing is, in its way, tried and true, because these are the organizations that I know best, the books that I own and have (except for all four volumes of one particular book) read and reread, the pharmacies from whom I order my own remedies.

As this book has been the truth of homeopathy as I understand it, this list is what I can recommend to you as a grouping of resources that can take you far beyond anything I have to offer.

BOOKS ABOUT HOMEOPATHY

This is only a brief list of books available on subjects related to homeopathy, so I have tried to select those that I have found, over the years, to be of the most value to me. Within each category below, I have started the list with the one or two books that I consider to be the finest of that category and have worked down from there.

The Organon

Organon of the Medical Art by Samuel Hahnemann, M.D. Edited and annotated by Wenda Brewster O'Reilly, Ph.D.; translated by Steven Decker. Palo Alto, CA: Birdcage Press (reprint edition: 2001). Simply the best. This is the one translation of the *Organon* that should be on your bookshelf. Nothing else comes close. (I also suggest that you buy the hardback edition, because you will refer to this book again and again over the years.)

Organon of Medicine by Samuel Hahnemann, M.D. Translated and with a preface by William Boericke, M.D. New Delhi: B. Jain Publishers (reprint edition: 2002). This is the cheapest edition of the *Organon* available today. It is sort of a mongrel edition, with no editor, no apparent guiding hand. But it presents the sixth edition of Hahnemann's work in adequate translation and is a good, simple edition for the home bookshelf.

Repertories

Repertory of the Homeopathic Materia Medica with Word Index by James Tyler Kent, M.D. New Delhi: B. Jain Publishers (reprint edition: 2002). This is the classic, basic Repertory written by American homeopath J. T. Kent. It belongs on the bookshelf of every student of homeopathy. It is very complete, very basic. Every other homeopath since Kent has based his Repertory on this pioneering work.

Homeopathic Medical Repertory, A Modern Alphabetical Repertory by Robin Murphy, N.D. Pagosa Springs, CO: Hahnemann Academy of North America (reprint edition: 2005). I really like this particular Repertory, as it is organized in alphabetical order (many others, including Kent's operate from the top of the head to the bottom of the feet, making it difficult at times to find the listings for the part of the body you are researching). As a modern Repertory, it also has rubrics for conditions and situations that were unknown two hundred years ago.

Synthesis Repertorium by Frederik Schroyens, M.D. London: Homeopathic Book Publishers (1993). *The Synthesis,* as it is known, is one of the most commonly used Repertories today. As the name implies, this work pulls together symptoms rubrics from several sources, making it the largest, if not the most complete Repertory published in a single volume. Because of the cost of this work, as well as its complexity, this Repertory is most often to be found in the office of medical professionals and not on the home bookshelf.

The Complete Repertory by Roger Van Zandvoort. Leidschendam, Netherlands: IRHIS Publishers (reprint edition: 1996). It certainly lives up to its name. It is very complete, very detailed. I personally believe that it could be a bit more user friendly in its format, but it delivers an extraordinary amount of information.

Materia Medicas

Pocket Manual of Homeopathic Materia Medica by William Boericke, M.D. New Delhi: B. Jain Publishers (reprint edition: 2003). It may seem to be a case of damning something with faint praise, but this volume is in so many homes because this is the cheapest of all the Materia Medicas. It is far from the most complete, but it is a basic, helpful book. It should be further noted that when Boericke's Materia Medica was first published it was not particularly well thought of, but it has become the basic and omnipresent Materia Medica of the modern age. Worth owning, but serious students should not only own this one.

Concordant Materia Medica by Frans Vermeulen. Haarlem, Netherlands: Merlijn Publishers (reprint edition: 1994). This is probably the Materia Medica that I use most often, in that it combines the notes of classical homeopaths Boericke, Phatak, Boger, Lippe, Allen, Pulford, Cowperthwaite, Kent, and Clarke with Vermeulen's own observations into a wonderful single volume Materia Medica of astounding richness and depth. I highly recommend this book.

Lotus Materia Medica by Robin Murphy, N.D. Pagosa Springs, CO: Lotus Star Academy (1995). This was created as a companion volume to Murphy's excellent Repertory. While the Materia Medica is riddled with typographical errors and some issues of clarity that may have been corrected in future editions, his unique take on the remedies and their uses makes this a solid addition to any homeopathic research library.

Desktop Guide to Keynotes and Confirmatory Symptoms by Roger Morrison, M.D. Grass Valley, CA: Hahnemann Clinic Publishing (1993). I really like this book and find it of value again and again. This is a modern Materia Medica and is a bit different from the others. It is not meant to be an exhaustive listing of all remedies and listings, instead it is a practical look at the remedies that are most commonly used and the guiding symptoms of each.

The Guiding Symptoms of Our Materia Medica by Constantine Hering, M.D. New Delhi: B. Jain Publishers (reprint edition: 1997). If you want the complete Materia Medica, you might want to spring for this one. It takes Hering ten volumes to work his way through the complete list of homeopathic remedies, but this reference work is excellent and well worth the investment.

Systematic Materia Medica of Homeopathic Remedies with Totality of Characteristic Symptoms and Various Indications of Each Remedy by K.N. Mathur. New Delhi: B. Jain Publishers (1988). This book may be difficult for you to get a hold of, but it is well worth the effort. Not a complete Materia Medica, but a book dedicated to the study of the most commonly used homeopathic remedies. Because of Mathur's unique take on the remedies—one steeped in homeopathy as it is practiced in India—I often turn to this volume when studying the remedies.

Materia Medica Pura (two volumes) by Samuel Hahnemann, M.D. New Delhi: B. Jain Publishers (reprint edition: 1986). What was, in its time, the first homeopathic Materia Medica is, today, far from the best. The book contains Hahnemann's notes on some sixty-odd remedies, ranging from polycrests such as Sulphur and Lycopodium, to odd remedies that have been lost in the two hundred-plus years of homeopathic practice. I find the book to be of little value in understanding or using the remedies. It is, however, of unique historic interest.

Drug Pictures by Margaret Tyler. Saffron Walden, England: C. W. Daniel (1952). This volume is a rather delightful trip into the mind of British homeopath Margaret Tyler. As sort of a combination Materia Medica and personal memoir, it is a unique volume and one that is not only very interesting to read, but also extremely educational in its content. This book is highly recommended.

Lectures on Homeopathic Materia Medica by James Tyler Kent, M.D. New Delhi: B. Jain Publishers (reprint edition: 1986). It is sort of cheating to list this book in this category, because it is not a true Materia Medica. Sadly, Kent never wrote one. Instead, the lectures that he gave his students on the various homeopathic remedies have been grouped together in this volume. While it is not the sort of book that you can quickly use to confirm a symptom, it is a valuable study of many of our most-used remedies.

Books about Homeopathy

Lectures on Homeopathic Philosophy by James Tyler Kent, M.D. Berkeley: North Atlantic Books (reprint edition: 1979). For my money, when it comes to learning about the practice of homeopathy as it is meant to be practiced, it all comes down to the work of two men—Hahnemann and Kent. This book is essential to the understanding of the philosophy of homeopathic medicine and the ramifications of its practice. A must-have book.

The Science of Homeopathy by George Vithoulkas. New York: Grove Press (1980). When it was first published, this was a groundbreaking work, in that it considered homeopathy from the scientific point of view. In that modern science had broken the boundaries of what had been, heretofore, the invisible aspects of nature, Vithoulkas, by considering homeopathy through the prism of (then) modern physics, makes a powerful statement of just how and why homeopathy works. Now, over a quarter century later, the book has taken on a retro aspect, but is still worth the reading.

Psyche and Substance: Essays on Homeopathy in the Light of Jungian Psychology by Edward C. Whitmont, M.D. Berkeley: North Atlantic Books (1991). If I were to say flat out that this is one of the best books ever written on the subject of homeopathy, I might be revealing my own personal bias, but I would also be stating simple fact. No other homeopath of my acquaintance ever impressed me as Whitmont did. His viewpoint is unique and his writing is excellent.

The Alchemy of Healing: Psyche and Soma by Edward C. Whitmont, M.D. Berkeley: North Atlantic Books (1993). If possible, this is even a better book than his first. Whitmont was one of the best writers ever to deal with topics related to homeopathy. And this book is Whitmont writing at the top of his game.

Divided Legacy: A History of the Schism in Medical Thought (4 volumes) by Harris Coulter. Berkeley: North Atlantic Books (1975, 1977, 1981, 1994). Let's face it, to tell the truth, this book, like Proust's *Remembrance of Things Past,* is one of those books that we all buy, but none of us read. We try and try, but we never get through the four volumes. What you do make it through, however, will enlighten you as to the history of homeopathy in the United States, and how it went from a thriving medical practice to a fringe alternative medicine.

The Patient, Not the Cure: The Challenge of Homoeopathy by Margery Blackie, M.D. Santa Barbara: Woodbridge Press (1978). Blackie's viewpoint can be best summed up with her brief phrase: "Homeopathy is not a philosophy, it is a principle." Her book reminds us that homeopathic medicine is based upon an immutable foundation and that its practice, therefore, should always adhere to the Laws of Cure. The title reminds us of just what it is that makes homeopathic medicine so difficult to practice—the fact that we are always and forever treating people, and never their diseases. As the book (and an amusing photograph inside the cover) reminds us, Blackie once served as the physician to Britain's Queen Elizabeth II, back when that was something to brag about.

A Dictionary of Homeopathic Medical Terminology by Jay Yasgur. Greenville, PA: Van Hoy Publishers (1992). This little book will be of great help to you, as it acts as a bridge between the arcane medical jargon used in many Repertories and Materia Medicas and the English language as it is spoken today. It also supplies brief biographical sketches of those who shaped the practice of homeopathy.

Home Guides

Practical Homeopathy by Vinton McCabe. New York: St. Martin's Press (2000). I swear that my editor made me list my own home guides here in this resource list, but I am truly proud of this book. I worked hard to not only give a working Materia Medica for the fifty remedies most commonly used in household emergencies, but also to flesh out the practice of homeopathy as it applies to acute situations. This book is based upon twenty year's worth of my own notes and observations.

Household Homeopathy by Vinton McCabe. Laguna Beach, CA: Basic Health Publications (2005). After having taught my final class on the practice of homeopathy, a year-long in-depth course in acute treatments for those who wanted to move beyond the information contained in most basic classes and home guides, I fleshed out my notes into this book, which stresses the use of objective symptoms in the selection of remedies. This book is largely based upon the writings of American homeopath John Scudder.

Homeopathic Medicine at Home: Natural Remedies for Everyday Ailments and Minor Injuries by Maesimund B. Panos, M.D. and Jane Heimlich. Los Angeles: J. P. Tarcher (reprint edition: 1981). This was the first homeopathic home guide that I ever owned and was the book that has launched so many others in the modern age. Panos and Heimlich looked back to a time over a hundred years ago, when many homeopaths published little volumes of suggested remedies for home use. They took this information into a new century and with information relating to the American home and family. This is still one of the best home guides and one of the easiest to use.

The Family Guide to Homeopathy: Symptoms and Natural Solutions by Andrew Lockie, M.D. New York: Simon & Schuster/Fireside (1993). I've always really liked this exhaustive work by a British practitioner. Lockie takes almost a naturopathic approach to home healthcare in this book, and gives not only the suggested homeopathic remedies to choose from, but also important rules for first aid and other "non-homeopathic" information.

The Complete Homeopathy Handbook by Miranda Castro. New York: St. Martin's Press (reprint edition: 1991). The subtitle says it all: "Safe and Effective Ways to Treat Fevers, Coughs, Colds and Sore Throats, Childhood Ailments, Food Poisoning, Flu, and a Wide Range of Everyday Complaints." In what is her best book, in my opinion, Castro gives good insight into the remedies that are most commonly associated with the included maladies. She is particularly good at including important emotional and mental symptoms.

Homeopathy for Pregnancy, Birth, and Your Baby's First Year by Miranda Castro. New York, St. Martin's Griffin (1993). While I am not a woman and have no children, I can still recognize that Miranda Castro writes about subjects related to homeopathy with a warmth and humor all too often missing from these books. This excellent guide lives up to its title, giving exhaustive information on the issues surrounding pregnancy and birth, as well as post-natal care and early childhood healthcare.

For other books related to women's health and childbirth, consider: *The Woman's Guide to Homeopathy* by Andrew Lockie, M.D. and Nicola Geddes. New York: St. Martin's Press (1994); *Natural Healing for Women: Caring for Yourself with Herbs, Homeopathy, and Essential Oils* by Susan Curtis and Romy Fraser. Rochester, VT: Thorson's Publishing (reprint edition: 2003); and *Homeopathic Medicine for Pregnancy and Childbirth* by Richard Moskowitz. Berkeley: North Atlantic Books (1992).

Poisons That Heal by Eileen Nauman. Flagstaff, AZ: Light Technology Publishing (1997). This isn't really a home guide, unless, of course, you are dealing with cases of Ebola in your own home. But Nauman's book is the sort of thing that I like best—one that presents homeopathic remedies in their widest range of uses. One that does not shy away from any topic related to homeopathy. This is really one of my favorite homeopathic books.

INTERNET RESOURCES

There now seem to be an endless number of websites dedicated to homeopathy and related alternative medicines. Some give great information, while others are questionable at best. In the list that follows, I offer some web addresses for the sites that I have found to be the best and most reliable. Rather than offer sites that cover the same ground over and over again, I have elected to give you the best site in each "category," meaning that I have offered the best site for helping you find a practitioner, the best of ordering books or remedies, the best for downloading articles, and so forth.

www.homeopathyhome.com: Without a doubt, this is the single best and most comprehensive site on the Internet on the subject of homeopathy. From here, you can link to virtually every other site and research the topic of homeopathy from A to Z. Everything is well organized and laid out, making this site very user friendly. Further, you can download any number of books and articles about homeopathy from this site, even a free copy of the *Organon*.

www.holisticmed.com/www/homeopathy.html: Use this address to find links to just about anything you can think of pertaining to homeopathy that has an online presence. International links to study groups, organizations, schools, pharmacies, and more are well organized and up to date. Bookmark this site for regular use.

www.homeopathic.org: This is the home page of the National Center for Homeopathy, one of our nation's largest homeopathic organizations. In addition to information specific to that organization, this site is very helpful for locating homeopathic practitioners across the United States.

www.lyghtforce.com: This is the home site for the Lyghtforce online discussion group. From this site, you can join the group and access archives of past discussions. This group offers solid information on homeopathy for both medical professionals and laypeople.

www.lyghtforce.com/homeopathyonline: This is the address for access to the Internet journal Homeopathy Online. This journal gives excellent information on the latest discoveries concerning homeopathy and case studies of its practice.

www.webhomeopath.com: Offers an online resource for repertorization. Several standard repertories are available for database search. Web Homeopath offers both free-trial memberships and full-service paid memberships.

www.homeoint.org: Website of the French organization Homéopathe International. This site is filled with valuable information about homeopathy and contains numerous books and articles online. Of special interest is the number of Materia Medicas offered online for search and study.

www.baltimore-homeopathy.org: This is the website of the powerful and organized Baltimore study group. This excellent site is made all the more impressive by the fact that it is a volunteer effort. Site contains solid information on homeopathy, and its study and practice.

www.julianwinston.com: This is the web page of the late teacher and historian Julian Winston. In his life, he was without peer as an educator and as the keeper of the flame for the history and development of homeopathy. In many ways, this site is his legacy. It contains a treasure trove of homeopathic information.

www.minimum.com: Home page for Minimum Priced Books, perhaps the best and most comprehensive of all the online resources for books on homeopathy. If there is a homeopathic Amazon.com, this is it.

www.homeopathyovernight.com: In my opinion, this is the best online service for ordering homeopathic remedies. The staff knows their stuff and the remedies come as the name promises—overnight. Orders may also be placed by calling 1-800-ARNICA3 (276-4223).

HOMEOPATHIC ORGANIZATIONS

National Center for Homeopathy (NCH)
801 North Fairfax Street, Suite #306
Alexandria, VA 22314
1-877-624-0613
www.homeopathic.org
This is the most polarizing of all homeopathic organizations. Some members of the homeopathic community think that it is the best of all the organizations, others wouldn't touch it with a ten-foot pole. For my part, I let my membership lapse years ago and would never consider returning. In past years, before the Internet opened up the flow of information on homeopathy and the possibility for global classrooms, the NCH held tight on its control over homeopathic education, deciding which classes laypeople could and could not attend. The fact that they are supported by the membership dollars of lay people, but have so little respect for them has always left a bad taste in my mouth.

The American Institute of Homeopathy (AIH)
801 North Fairfax Street, Suite # 306
Alexandria, VA 22314
1-888-445-9988
www.homeopathyusa.org
Our nation's oldest homeopathic organization, the AIH is a professional organization with memberships available only to medical doctors, doctors of osteopathy, podiatrists, and dentists who make use of homeopathics in their practice, or who are supportive of homeopathy in general. The organization publishes a quarterly journal *The Journal of the American Institute of Homeopathy* and supports educational and research efforts in the field of homeopathy. The AIH is especially supportive to physicians who are newly establishing their homeopathic practice.

North American Society of Homeopaths
P.O. Box 450039
Sunrise, FL 33345
(206) 720-7000
www.homeopathy.org
Another organization of professional homeopaths, although, as far as I am concerned, this one has never quite gotten its act together. Publishes a magazine called *The American Homeopath*.

Homeopathic Academy of Naturopathic Physicians
P.O. Box 8341
Covington, WA 98042
(253) 630-3338
www.hanp.net
This organization is open only to naturopathic physicians who incorporate homeopathy into their practice. They publish a professional journal. Perhaps their most
important function is that they certify naturopathic physicians in the practice of
homeopathy. This allows those of us who visit a certified practitioner to know that
they have met with a standard of education and excellence.

Foundation for Homeopathic Education and Research
2124 Kittredge Street
Berkeley, CA 94704
(510) 649-0294
www.homeopathic.com
This one is a bit confusing. The Foundation for Homeopathic Education and Research is the not-for-profit wing of Homeopathic Educational Services, a for-profit
supplier of tapes, books, software and remedies, located at the same address (see next
page). The foundation supports research in the field of homeopathy and sponsors lectures and classes on the same. Both aspects of the business are under the firm control
of homeopathic author and educator Dana Ullman.

HOMEOPATHIC PHARMACEUTICAL FIRMS
AND PHARMACIES

All those listed below sell homeopathic remedies, some by kit, some by single remedies, most by both. Many of these businesses also supply other homeopathic products
as well, from books to tapes to software. All those listed below are recognized for
meeting all the standards for the creation and storage of homeopathic products
and can be well trusted as remedy sources. Note that some of the businesses listed here
supply only remedies, others sell books, tapes, and so forth, along with the remedies.

Boericke & Tafel
1375 North Mountain Springs Parkway
Springville, UT 84663
1-800-962-8873
Although they have no dedicated website, their remedies can be ordered online
through a number of sources.

Boiron-Bornemann, Inc.
6 Campus Boulevard, Building A
Newtown Square, PA 19073
Also:
98 C. West Cochran Street
Simi Valley, CA 93065
1-800-258-8823
www.boiron.com

Dolisos, America, Inc.
3014 Rigel Road
Las Vegas, NV 89102
(702) 871-7153
www.lyghtforce.com/dolisos

Homeopathic Educational Services
2124 Kittredge Street
Berkeley, CA 94704
1-800-359-9051
www.homeopathic.com

Homeopathy Overnight
929 Shelburne Avenue
Absecon, NJ 08201
1-800-ARNICA3 (276-4223)
www.homeopathyovernight.com

Luyties Pharmacal Company
P.O. Box 8080
Richford, VT 05476
1-800-HOMEOPATHY (466-3672)
www.1800homeopathy.com

Similasan Corporation
1745 Shea Center Drive, Suite 380
Highlands Ranch, CO 80129
1-800-426-1644
www.similasan.com

Standard Homeopathic Company
204-210 West 131st Street
Los Angeles, CA 90061
1-800-624-9659
www.hylands.com
Standard now also own and operates Hyland's, Inc., another homeopathic pharmaceutical firm. For more information on both companies, go to website listed here.

Washington Homeopathic Products
33 Fairfax Street
Berkeley Springs, WV 25411
1-800-336-1695
www.homeopathyworks.com

Index

About the Author

Vinton McCabe is the author of six books on the subject of health and healing. Most notably, he is the author of several books on the subject of homeopathy, including *Homeopathy, Healing & You* (1998) and *Practical Homeopathy* (2000), both published by St. Martin's Press. Most recently, he is the author of *Household Homeopathy*, published in January of 2005 by Basic Health Publications. He is also the co-author, with Dr. Marc Grossman, of *Greater Vision*, a book on natural vision improvement, which was published in 2002 by Keats Publishing.

He has studied homeopathy for the past twenty-five years, and served as a homeopathic educator for the past fifteen. He also served as the president of the Connecticut Homeopathic Association from the establishment of that non-profit organization in 1985 until his move to rural Connecticut in the year 2000. As the chief educator for that organization, he has been responsible for training thousands of laypeople and medical professionals alike in the basics of homeopathic philosophy and in the proper uses of homeopathic remedies.

In addition, McCabe has served on the faculty both of the Open Center of Manhattan and the Wainwright House of Rye, New York as a homeopathic educator. He also taught homeopathy at the Learning Annex, the Omega Institute, the New York Botanical Garden, and the Seminar Center in Manhattan. He also served as a member of the Board of Directors for the Hudson Valley School for Classical Homeopathy, for whom he also developed educational materials. He also traveled throughout the United States, teaching courses in homeopathic philosophy and the uses of homeopathic and Bach flower remedies.

Vinton McCabe is presently at work on a series of three new books for Basic Health Publications on the subjects of homeopathy, Bach flower remedies, and cell salts. He is also at work on a book on moderating high blood pressure through natural treatments.

McCabe has worked with medical professionals, including acupuncturists, naturopaths, and chiropractors, as a homeopathic consultant. He also is a trained vision therapist, and practiced vision therapy for seven years (1993–2000) at the Rye Learning Center in Rye, New York.

In addition to his work in vision therapy and homeopathy, Vinton McCabe has won awards for his journalism, as well as for poetry and theatrical writing. He is a published novelist. Recently, he was awarded an individual artist grant by the Connecticut Commission on the Arts for the creation of his first full-length drama, "Appassionata." In 1990, he was given the Dewar's Young Artist award in poetry.

Vinton McCabe has also worked as a producer, a writer, and a host in both television and radio. He was producer and host of the PBS series *Artsweek*, and creator and executive producer of *Healthplan*, an award-winning health-care special produced by Connecticut Public Television. On radio, he has acted as a film and theater critic and hosted his own daily talk show.

As a print journalist, Vinton McCabe has done features work for many weekly and daily papers, as well as monthly publications, including *New England Monthly*, *The Stamford Advocate* and *The New York Times*.